THE **TAO** OF
LOVE

THE **TAO** OF

LOVE

by Cheng Heng

Translated from the French by Arthur Denner

MARLOWE & COMPANY
NEW YORK

Published by
Marlowe & Company
632 Broadway, Seventh Floor
New York, NY 10012

Library of Congress Catalog Card Number 97-71757

ISBN 1-56924-817-6

Manufactured in the United States of America.

First Edition

Note

This book is based on traditional Chinese principles of health and cannot take the place of a medical consultation or professional medical advice. The traditional formulas and exercises are presented here for informational purposes only; neither the authors nor the publishers assume responsibility for their use or application.

CONTENTS

Introduction   page
  The Teachings of Master Cheng Heng   1

Chapter One
  The Male Sexual Tao   47

Chapter Two
  The Female Sexual Tao   101

Chapter Three
  The Nine Exercises of The Sexual Tao   131

Chapter Four
  Green Dragon and White Tiger: The Sexual Union   173

INTRODUCTION

The Teachings of
Master Cheng Heng

"The medicine is produced in the secret gateway;

The alchemical fire blazes up in the yang furnace;

When the Dragon and the Tiger are subdued,

The golden cup will yield forth the mystic pearl."

THE TAO OF LOVE

THIS BOOK presents the teachings of several Taiwanese Taoist masters under the collective pseudonym of Cheng Heng. The subject of these teachings is human sexuality, and the approach is a traditional one.

Unlike some books on the sexual Tao, this book presents Taoist methods in detail; it does not, however, like others, offer dangerous methods that, while useful for the committed Taoist, can only sow confusion in the mind of the Western reader.

With its traditional format and structure, this text has been written as a collection of teachings that the reader can consult as he or she pleases. However, certain terms have precise meanings that can be understood only if encountered by the reader in the order in which the book presents them; we therefore strongly advise an initial cover-to-cover reading.

Great care has gone into the preparation of this work; nonetheless, because the pages that follow represent traditional teachings drawn from the Chinese experience, the application and practice of these teachings, particularly those that concern recipes, herbal formulas, and exercises, are wholly the responsibility of the reader. The authors and editors assume no responsibility for the application of the teachings contained herein.

4

STRENGTHENING THE SEXUAL ENERGIES

Nearly two thousand years ago the Chinese philosopher Mencius said, "Hunger and sexual desire are both part of human nature." In the book *The Union of Yin and Yang*, it is written that "the sexual act allows vital energy and blood to circulate through the vital organs of the body." *The Book of Prescriptions* explains that "sexuality can be harmful or beneficial: those who know how to use it can protect their good health, whereas those who abuse it can die before their time."

The oldest of the treatises on sexuality, however, is the *Su Nu Jing* (The book of explanations about sexuality). It has been attributed to the mythical emperor Huangdi, who is also the reputed author of the *Neijing*, the Chinese medical classic. Taoists consider the *Su Nu Jing* the theoretical foundation of healthy sexual practices based on the balancing of yin and yang. This treatise, now more than two thousand years old, begins thus:

> The Yellow Emperor said to Su Nu, "I am tired, my entire being is out of balance. I am anxious from morning till night and can feel that my days are numbered. How did this happen?" And Su Nu answered, "This trouble is caused by an overall imbalance between your yin and your yang, resulting from inadequate sexual activity. If the woman is stronger, sexually speaking, the man will dissipate his forces and lose his

sexual vigor. This state resembles a fire that goes out when water is poured on it. Sex is like cooking: to get a tasty dish, it must be cooked just right, with only as much water and fire as are necessary. Similarly, one must experiment with the principle of the union of water and fire; in this way one can experience the right sexual pleasure. Otherwise, disharmony will result and your life will soon come to an end."

In ancient China, sexuality was considered an activity that could bring happiness or unhappiness, particularly in the area of human health. The key to a harmonious sex life lies in understanding the yin and yang energies of the universe, in achieving a balanced equilibrium between the passive and active forces that govern life and death.

Westerners tend to think of sexuality solely from the perspective of the immediate gratification it can offer, without trying to understand its energies and its physical, social, and spiritual implications.

Taoists, although sometimes reproved for having free morals, were nonetheless extremely careful and meticulous as far as energies were concerned. For Taoists, the sexual act is a serious matter that involves a man's and a woman's most intense energies. Making use of these fantastically powerful energies requires a thorough knowledge of the processes and forces that sexuality brings into play.

Sun Si-miao, a Taoist physician of the Tang dynasty period, was renowned for his medical expertise. He lived to be more than one hundred years old, an achievement generally attributed to his having followed the precise sexual prescriptions he gave others. These concerned the frequency of sexual relations—which, according to Sun Si, were to vary in accordance with a person's age—as well as techniques for making love.

Apart from their precepts having to do with sexual energies, Taoists also viewed male-female relations as a question of interpersonal harmony and understanding. As Su Nu advised the Yellow Emperor, "A happy and harmonious sexual life depends in large measure on there being harmony and understanding between the two partners."

Civilizations the world over have sensed the power of sexuality, and throughout the ages rulers have sought to control and sometimes repress many of its facets. The world's religions have weighed in with their views as well, and all of them have sought to exert some influence in the sexual domain. The twentieth century brought its ideas of sexual liberation to the world, but whatever sexual freedom men and women may enjoy today, they are often totally ignorant as to the workings of their sexual energies; more often than not, they are slaves to their pleasure rather than its masters.

For Taoists, sexuality is the root of life—what the ancients spoke of as vital essence, or *jing*, one of the "three treasures" (*san bao*). This *jing*, or sexual energy, is also the motor of human evolution, and because it can be transformed into spiritual energy, it can play an active role in the development of one's being. Squandering this precious energy during adolescence, young adulthood, or later in life can have grave repercussions on a person's physical and mental health.

The Taoists' first observation about sexuality was concerned with the proper frequency of relations according to a person's age and physical constitution. The ancient Taoists offered other advice as well, explaining how to carry out the sex act by coordinating it with breathing and with Taoist energy practices. For the most part, however, their teachings are concerned with strengthening the basic energies through special exercises.

The first piece of advice that Taoists would offer young men and women was to warn them of the dangers of beginning a sex life too early. The ancient Taoists compared the loss of sexual energy during youth to the weakening of a sapling's roots. One way of losing precious *jing* too early in life is by masturbating on a regular basis. Masturbation provides no opportunity for contact with the opposite sex; as a result, the two energies, yin and yang, cannot nourish each other and the young man or woman ends up losing some of his or her vital substance. In the *Treatise on Longevity*, it is said that "the opposition and union of yin and yang are the universal law of Nature." Young men can emit their semen at most twice a month. Regular masturbation directly affects the root of life, or *jing*. Practiced at a young age and on a regular basis, masturbation is all the more likely, in both sexes, to diminish longevity and weaken immunity.

In the *Su Nu Jing*, the legendary emperor receives the principles of a healthy sexuality from "a woman of knowledge." The first thing she teaches him is the value of the three treasures.

SAN BAO, OR THE THREE TREASURES

The three treasures, or *san bao*, form the basis of ancient Taoist energy work. Together they represent the human being's physical, spiritual, and energy potentials.

Anyone wishing to take the Taoist spiritual path must
first purify his or her physical energies and be in reasonably
good health. Similarly, to reap the benefits of a healthy and
vigorous sexuality, one's physical energies must be strong
and pure and one's spirit must be free from the disruptive
domination of the five senses and the seven emotions.

Before embarking on the practice of Taoist exercises and
methods for sexual strengthening, one needs to understand
the human being as an energy structure. The *san bao*, with
its tripartite model of the three treasures, offers the perfect
illustration of this structure. When a person keeps his body,
breathing, and consciousness in harmony, it is said that he
possesses the three treasures: *qi* (pronounced *chi*), *jing*, and
shen. These three treasures are nothing other than a new
subjective differentiation of cosmic energy. Lu Dong Bing
gives this precise and vivid description of them:

> *Jing* is the root of life, the body of flesh and blood. . . .
> *Qi* is vital energy, movement, activity, speech, and per-
> ception, the door of life and death. *Shen* [spiritual
> awareness] is the mind, the sparkle in the eyes, con-
> scious thought; it is wisdom and intelligence, intui-
> tion, and the potential for awakening.

Like any treasures, these three are not easily come by. The
key to developing them, and thus to achieving good health,
is tranquility and profound peace of mind, not excitement
and uncontrolled passions.

When grave or chronic illness occurs, the way to find
healing energy is not to deny or reject the illness but to
balance and develop the three treasures. Denial often
comes from fear or the feeling that the illness is unfair.

People tend to seek the causes of their illness in external factors and prefer not to recognize the extent to which their own lifestyles, habits, mind-sets, behaviors, and emotions are implicated in the state of their health. Nevertheless, all these factors are part of the three treasures: they are the uncut gem that needs to be worked on. This book offers a way of discovering the three treasures that is centered on sexuality; it presents simple practices that make use of all the facets of the Taoist healing tradition. These diverse facets use the different functions of the three treasures; that is why true healing cannot be based on a single point of view but must encompass the many faculties and potentials that all of us have within ourselves.

Acupuncture, herbal therapies, and massage are all good healing methods, but none of these therapies can claim to be a panacea any more than psychotherapy can. All that a holistic view of health such as that of the ancient Taoists can do is try to harness the resources of the three treasures: energy, body, and mind.

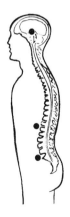

The three treasures represented symbolically in the body.

QI, OR VITAL MOBILE ENERGY

Qi, or breath-energy, is a fundamental concept of Chinese medicine. It is difficult to translate the full meaning of the Chinese character, which signifies energy in the form of steam that has accumulated in a pot of boiling water.

Qi is multiple in nature, and numerous Taoist treatises speak of a *qi* of nature, a *qi* of plants, a *qi* of fire, and a *qi* of water (hydraulic force). One might even compare it with the *prâna,* or vital breath, of Indian yogic and tantric theories.

Normal human *qi* is formed from inborn *qi (yuanqi),* which is transmitted to the child from the parents at the moment of conception. This *qi* is stored in the kidneys and the *mingmen,* or Vital Gate, which is associated with the suprarenal area or adrenal glands. The two other types of *qi,* which together make up acquired *qi,* are grain, or alimentary, *qi (guqi),* which comes from the digestion of food, and air *qi (gongqi),* which is extracted from the air through breathing.

Together, these three forms of *qi* produce the normal *qi* that permeates the entire body. According to traditional texts, *qi* has five main functions. It is the source of all bodily movements. All voluntary physical activities (walking, etc.) and involuntary movements (the heartbeat, etc.) are caused by *qi,* or vital energy. It circulates along the body's acupuncture channels and in the tissues. *Qi* protects the body from pathogenic atmospheric influences (cold, wind, humidity, and so on); it opens and closes the pores of the skin. *Qi* controls the transformation of substances in the body, keeping them in balance; it regulates flows and discharges of blood, urine, sweat, tears, and so on. *Qi* is responsible for keeping the body's organs and substances where they belong; it thus prevents collapses of organs, or ptoses, and excessive or untimely discharges of vital fluids (including sperm). Lastly, *qi* warms the body and, through the system known as the Triple Burner, maintains the body's economy of energy.

When a person's *qi* is sick, various symptoms appear. These symptoms are the kind often seen in today's medical practices. If a person has a deficiency of *qi*, he experiences lethargy and fatigue and lacks the desire to move. Deficiency of *qi* can also refer to a deficiency in a single organ (which, in the theory of the Five Evolutive Phases, is related to the five elements: wood, fire, earth, metal, and water) or to the deficiency of a certain type of *qi*, for example, protective *qi*. *Qi* deficiencies of this latter sort result in cold limbs, aversion to cold, and spontaneous sweating. If a person has sinking *qi*, *qi* descends and cannot hold the organs in place. Ptosis of the stomach and prolapse of the uterus are two examples of sinking *qi*. Stagnant *qi* has to do with obstructions of *qi* that give rise to aches and pains or paralyses. Dyspnea—that is, difficult or labored breathing, the feeling of the breath being blocked in the lungs—is an example of stagnant *qi*. Rebellious *qi*, a form of stagnant *qi*, is *qi* going in the wrong direction. Vomiting and belching are two examples of rebellious *qi*.

In the context of yin-yang theory, *qi* is, relatively speaking, an active substance and therefore associated with yang. Conversely, deficient *qi* is a yin-type condition of hypoactivity.

To simplify a little, one might say that within the human body there are several *qi* or energies at work: the hereditary energy that comes from our parents and is connected to the genital functions and the life capital that we receive at birth; and the acquired energy that we obtain from the combination of the foods we eat and the air we breathe. Acquired energy nourishes the internal organs and protects the body against attacks from its environment. Taoist health exercises work primarily on this energy, their goal being to fortify it. Together, hereditary energy and acquired energy constitute *zhengqi*, or original vitality.

Chinese health exercises and the sexual Tao are designed to help a person fortify *zhengqi* in a number of ways: by harmonizing the body and respiration; by concentrating on the *dantian* (see below) through the practice of conscious abdominal breathing; by mobilizing *qi*—making it ascend, descend, and open—and closing the energy points (the Doors of Jade) of the *dantian* in the *niwan* (head) and the *shanzhong* (chest); by making *qi* circulate in the abdominal region through the *dantian, mingmen* (between the kidneys), and *huiyin* (perineal region); by concentrating the mind and stimulating *qi* and sexual *jing*.

JING, OR ORIGINAL ESSENCE

Jing, or original essence, is the underlying basis of life. It is one of the three fundamental substances of Taoist psychophysiology, the others being *qi* and *shen*. Taoist alchemists referred to these three substances as the three treasures and believed that each of them had to be purified through the quest for enlightenment, a process that goes well beyond the bounds of medical practices aimed at balancing the energies. Energy equilibrium, they believed, was at all events a temporary state, because ultimately, when death came, the yin energies would separate from the yang energies, the forces of heaven from those of earth.

Jing is the vehicle for the sexual energy that gives matter its forms. In one sense, it functions as an encoded message, or program. In another, more general sense, *jing* is like the philosopher's stone: it gives form to emptiness.

Jing has two sources. Innate, or congenital, jing comes from our parents (and is therefore hereditary); postnatal, or acquired, *jing* is derived from the purification or sublimation of the food that we eat. Disharmonies of *jing* tend to affect an individual's strength and the expression of his sexuality and are also implicated in male and female infertility.

Jing is situated in the lower cinnabar field or the Palace of the Yellow Court and the Vital Gate (*mingmen*). The kidneys are the organs that control *jing*. In relation to blood, which nourishes *jing* in its postnatal form, *jing* is yang. According to the *Su Wen*, one of the two books that constitute the *Neijing*, *jing* "is the quintessence, the origin of life."

As noted earlier, this biological substance governs all developmental processes—procreation, growth, maturation, decline, and death. *Jing* is the primary material substrate that exists before yin and yang and produces life with its subsequent differentiation into yin and yang. *Jing* is also considered the basic potential energy for producing vital activity, the continual process by which yin and yang are generated in the body's cells, tissues, and organs.

To function normally, the entire body and all its essential organs require *jing*. The energy necessary for initiating and maintaining the different body functions is concentrated in the kidneys. Thus the activity of each organ's yin and yang depends in the first instance on the yin and yang of the kidneys, because the kidneys are a reservoir of *jing*. The kidneys are also called "the residence of yin and yang," the origin of the yin and yang organs.

Innate *jing*

Innate *jing* is the quintessential substance received from our parents. Ling Shu says that "the beginning of life resides in *jing*; and because it is hereditary, it is called innate *jing*." Innate *jing* thus corresponds to the primordial life principle, the genetic inheritance contained in the egg and the sperm. It is what makes conception possible.

A person begins life with a determinate store of innate *jing* that diminishes qualitatively and quantitatively over the course of a lifetime because the kidneys are always nourishing the body's vital functions. One's level of *jing* declines with age. How quickly or slowly *jing* will be used up depends on one's hygiene and the diseases or accidents one meets with over the course of one's life.

Acquired *jing*

Acquired *jing* is accumulated after birth. It comes from the purification of foods into their essences in the course of digestion. Like innate *jing*, acquired *jing* is located in the kidneys, and it is just as indispensable to the vital functions: its task is to take over from innate *jing*, which would otherwise be used up much more quickly, thus diminishing the possibility of a long life. According to the medical classics, "The *jing* that we acquire over the course of our lives becomes the *jing* of the five viscera and the six bowels." *Jing* thus participates actively in the life process.

SHEN, OR AWARENESS, SPIRIT, MIND

Whereas *jing* is the source of life and *qi* makes it possible for us to move or to set things in motion, *shen* is conscious vitality. *Shen* represents the mirror of consciousness that can either be manifested in one of the seven emotions (anger, joy, sadness, grief, pensiveness, fear, and fright) or be purified in the beatific and empty state of objectless contemplation. Certain Chinese classic texts on Taoist spirituality say, through the mouth of the legendary Yellow Emperor, "Nourishing *shen* is the supreme task; nourishing the body is useful, but secondary." Nourishing *shen* through emptiness is one of the root ideas of Taoism. As the Taoist master of the dark secrets of heaven observed:

> To make your awareness like the sun that illuminates the world, try to generate a light akin to that of the Cosmic Emptiness. For *shen*, the mirror of emptiness, is composed of the original *qi* of heaven (inborn *qi*). At the beginning of things, there existed neither the intellect nor the perversion of the senses.

In the present context, however, *shen* should be understood as the reflection of vitality, consciousness, and the seven conflictual emotions. The light of *shen* can be seen in the gleam of the eyes, particularly in the pupils.

Signs of disturbed *shen* include incoherent thoughts and speech, a nearly total lack of luster in the eyes, insomnia, and frequent forgetfulness. Extreme disharmony of *shen* can lead to madness.

The Chinese medical classic, the *Neijing*, says,

The union of the two *jings* produces *shen*. The energy that circulates with *shen* is called *hun* (soul), the energy that circulates with *jing* is called *po*. That which commands all of this together is called heart, and the heart's memory is thought; decisive thought is determination.

In the theory of the Five Evolutive Phases, *hun* is associated with the liver, *po* with the lungs, and determination, or will, with the kidneys.

Jing and *qi* are both stored in the kidneys, which also control the bones and the production of marrow. The kidneys are the root of *qi*. Taoist sexual practices are useful for exercising, nourishing, and preserving *jing* and especially for exercising the vital energy contained in the kidneys.

In the practice of *qigong*, much attention is paid to preserving and training *shen*. That is why *qigong* masters have developed exercises to nourish the heart *(xin)* and calm, regulate, and preserve *shen*. Other disciplines too can help to regulate the body and breathing and harmonize the functions of the heart. These practices transform the activity of the brain and allow the body to feel relaxed and at ease; such a state is known as internal peace or *neiyang gong*. In this state, the body's metabolism slows down and oxygen consumption decreases as the storing of *qi* increases. The entire body's functioning is thereby directly affected and strengthened, and a state of disharmony gradually transforms into one of dynamic equilibrium.

Jing, qi, and *shen* play an important role in vital activity. Ancient Taoists and Chinese physicians, experts in preventive health care, accorded a special place to the use of exercise and Taoist meditation in conserving these three fundamental substances, particularly in the sexual domain.

The three treasures, *jing*, *qi*, and *shen*, exist only in their interdependence. They work together in the body and cannot be artificially dissociated. The body's health and longevity depend on the care that is taken to preserve *jing*, *qi*, and *shen*. The methods for transforming the three treasures follow the traditional schema indicated below:

METHOD	PRINCIPLE	RESULT
Manifest energy	Transform *jing* into *qi*	Strengthening of the bones
Hidden energy	Transform *qi* into *shen*	Strengthening of the sinews
Transmuted energy	Transform *shen* into emptiness	Strengthening of the marrow

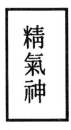

Ideograms of the three treasures.

THE SEXUAL TAO'S DOORS OF JADE

Before undertaking any of the exercises in this book, it is necessary to have an idea of the ancient Taoists' conception of the anatomical energies, in particular, some important points where *qi* is concentrated in the body. These essential points were called the Doors of Jade by certain ancient Taoist schools, which sought to emphasize how precious these points were for self-knowledge. They are intimately linked to sexuality and sexual energy.

THE ABDOMINAL CINNABAR FIELD, OR *XIA DANTIAN*

The term *dantian*, or cinnabar field, refers to three important zones that are traditionally associated with the three treasures: the upper cinnabar field, in the center of the head (*shen*); the middle cinnabar field, in the middle of the chest (*qi*); and the lower cinnabar field, in the center of the belly (*jing*).

The lower *dantian* is approximately four thumb widths below the navel, at a location corresponding roughly to the acupuncture point CV4 (Conception Vessel 4), a point known to acupuncturists as the sea of energy. It is a main focus for the meditative internal-healing practices of *nei-yang gong* and is thought to be the site in the body where *qi* is generated and develops. All Chinese acupuncture and health-exercise traditions concur that concentrating thought and sensorial awareness on this point increases energy and improves a person's physical constitution. Certain ancient Taoist texts claim that diseases of all types can be cured through sustained concentration on this point.

The middle *dantian (zhanzong)*, known as the heart cavity or the scarlet palace, is level with the acupuncture point CV17, exactly midway between the nipples. This center is linked to heart energy, which in traditional Chinese medicine is connected with the functioning of spirit and consciousness. Women are sometimes advised to concentrate on this point, particularly during their menstrual periods, and so are adolescents; it helps eliminate obstructions of *qi* in the lower *dantian*.

The upper *dantian (yingtang)*, located between the eyebrows and level with acupuncture point GV24 (Governing Vessel 24), is also called the marvelous point, or *niwan*. It is used to treat many afflictions, including headaches, vertigo, disorders involving the eye and the nose, insomnia, convulsions, hypertonia, and tension. It is also used as a measuring point in cranial acupuncture.

From the standpoint of sexuality, it is extremely important for the abdominal cinnabar field to be strong and filled with energy. The word *tian* means "field." The *xia dantian* is not a particular point but a large zone. It is also called *qihai* (sea of energy) or *shenlu*, which means "crucible of consciousness." It is traversed by a number of channels: *Ren* (conception), *Chong*, kidney, stomach, liver, and spleen. The ancient Taoists called the *xia dantian* "the place where the five *qis* of the five viscera returned to their origin." The abdominal cinnabar field is thus an essential point for energy development. It is here that energy purified through *qigong* work is stored and concentrated. This essential and purified *qi*, the *zhengqi* of the body's organs and energy channels, concentrates in the abdominal *dantian*.

The *xia dantian* is an area that promotes the production, concentration, and circulation of *zhengqi* throughout the body. It does this by transforming *jing* into *qi* (as described above), by regulating and strengthening *qi*, by preserving *jing*, by fortifying the kidneys, spleen, and stomach, by toning the *Chong* channel and the uterus, and by warming the "palace of *jing*." The energy that collects at the *mingmen* (see below) between the two kidneys (the primordial *qi* of the

Triple Burner channel) flows into the abdominal *dantian* through special connections between the channels.

A traditional Taoist precept, "Focus your spirit on the point of *qi*," underscores the importance of the *xia dantian* in the process of energy transformation. According to oral Taoist traditions, the *xia dantian* is the crucible where the energies of heaven and earth come together, the site where earthly sustenance (food and drink) joins with the subtle breath of the universe through natural abdominal breathing. The breath, thus enriched, then circulates according to the well-known Taoist cycle of the Five Movements: first toward the liver, then toward the heart, spleen, and lungs, and finally to the kidneys. The *xia dantian* is thus the concrete basis of the Taoist sexual method.

Qihai, the Sea of Energy

Located one and a half thumb widths below the navel, this point is one of the external manifestations of the *xia dantian*. Chinese physicians consider it the stimulation point for *qi* in men. The sea of energy is also the area where the *zhenqi*, the primordial breath, is concentrated. Many Far Eastern practices rely on the *xia dantian* as the starting point for various kinds of energy work that involve such methods as massage, breathing, *qigong* poses, and Tai Chi Chuan. These practices regard the *qihai* point as the place where breath is produced. Taoist natural abdominal-breathing techniques refer to this point explicitly as the origin of breath.

The activation of this point has many positive effects on health and sexuality: it awakens the vital forces, dispels pathogenic abdominal cold, and stimulates kidney energy. The *qihai* and the *guanyuan*, which is discussed below, rep-

THE TAO OF LOVE

resent the two aspects of the cinnabar field: the *qihai* is the dynamic aspect, whereas the *guanyuan* plays a stabilizing role and helps develop groundedness.

Guanyuan: The Door of Ancestral Qi

This point is located in the middle of the abdomen, below the *qihai* point, exactly four thumb widths below the navel. It is the closest point on the outside of the body to the *xia dantian*; because of this proximity, it is traditionally held to be the external manifestation of the cinnabar field. In Chinese medicine, this point is the intersection of the three yin channels of the foot (the kidney channel, the liver channel, and the spleen channel) and also the point of origin of the autoregulatory system known as the Triple Burner (*sanjiao*). In Taoist energy work, this point is one of the most important for strengthening body and mind.

This point is used in traditional Chinese medicine in the treatment of yin and yang deficiencies, especially chronic illnesses. Its nourishing and toning action on energy and blood permits the stabilization of the emotions that practitioners of *qigong* are familiar with. When stabilization occurs, it is said that the spirit has been calmed by the action of the *guanyuan*. This point is particularly effective in reducing anxieties and grounding the etheric body.

THE *MINGMEN*, OR DOOR OF DESTINY

The *mingmen*, important to sexuality, is located between the two kidneys. *Mingmen* means "Vital Gate" or "Door of Destiny." It concentrates energy from the "anterior heaven," in other words, the vital hereditary energy of the kidneys. The *mingmen* is located in the small of the back, along the *Du* channel (governing vessel), between the kidneys. It is located exactly below the second lumbar vertebra, behind the navel. Some Taoists refer to it as the posterior *dantian*, because of its connection with the *xia dantian* (see above). According to the ancient treatise, the *Nan Jing*, the *mingmen* governs the kidneys. Located exactly between the kidneys, it permits communication among the kidneys, navel, heart, lungs, and brain. It is the source of vitality and the controller of the *"xiang* fire"—the fire of the Vital Gate—and the Elixir Field.

The *mingmen* is also a sea of *jing* and blood, just as the spleen and stomach are seas of water and food, respectively. Both serve as the foundation of the five viscera, or *zang* organs, because it is through them alone that the yin *qi* and yang *qi* of the five viscera are generated and develop. Whereas the *mingmen* is associated with the element fire, the kidneys, which are closely linked to the *mingmen*, are associated with water.

From the standpoint of their interaction, it is fire that directs water, because water is at the origin of fire. Water and fire are mutually dependent, each sustaining the other. They cannot be separated. The water of the kidneys and the fire of the *mingmen* are called primordial yin and primordial yang, respectively. Together, they constitute congenital *jing qi*. When primordial yin and yang are regulated and in balance, they can regulate and balance the yin and yang of the entire body.

The *mingmen* point is also important in *moxibustion*, the traditional Chinese medical technique that involves applying heat to the body by burning substances at some distance from the skin. A number of sexual deficiencies, including impotence and nocturnal emissions, can be treated by toning this point.

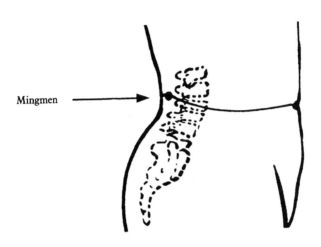

The mingmen *point.*

HUIYIN, THE CENTER OF THE PERINEUM

This point, located at the center of the perineum, between the scrotum and anus in males and between the posterior vulva and anus in females, is the point of origin of the *Ren, Du,* and *Chong* channels. In *qigong* sexual training, it is the point through which abdominal energy travels toward the spinal column. It is located at a key point between the anterior *Ren* channel and the posterior *Du* channel. It was once called "the bottom of the ocean." In Taoist energy theory, it is considered the source of reproductive *jing* and is associated with the genital functions in both males and females. As one ancient text explains, "The point located an inch in front of *huiyin* is where *jing* collects in the man; in the woman, this place is the uterus."

Clinical data has demonstrated that stimulating the *xia dantian* together with the *mingmen* and *huiyin* can directly affect the secretions of the adrenal and pituitary glands as well as those of the gonads. This effect is described by Chinese medicine as a stimulation of the yin and yang kidneys. In Chinese medicine, the *huiyin* functions as a regulator of vital energy in the *Ren*, *Du*, and *Chong* channels; it can be used to treat seminal emissions, male impotence, and irregular menstrual periods. But because of its intimate location, it is hardly ever used.

The ancient Taoists and practitioners of *qigong* regarded the kidneys, *mingmen*, abdominal *dantian*, *qihai* point, and *huiyin* point together as a general energy center, a unit that commands and regulates the vital activity of the human body.

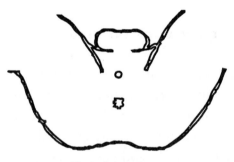

The huiyin *point.*

KIDNEY ENERGY AND SEXUALITY

The kidneys are located on both sides of the loins, or lumbar region, and are closely associated with the bladder, both functionally and by virtue of the connections between their respective acupuncture channels. Far Eastern medicine ascribes four important functions to the kidneys:

- Receiving hereditary energy and storing reproductive fluids. In modern medical language, this function is to be understood as referring to the connection between the adrenal hormones and sexual hormones.
- Producing spinal marrow, through the intermediary of the hormonal system (as above).
- Regulating the body's fluids through their metabolization. This function corresponds more closely to what modern medicine understands as the kidneys' activities.
- Regulating auditory functions. This connection between the ears and the kidneys means that latent kidney disorders can be diagnosed by identifying hearing problems (especially tinnitus, or ringing in the ears).

The language in which ancient Chinese medical doctrine is expressed may sometimes sound naive, but let there be no mistake: connections such as these offer proof that the Chinese physicians of yesteryear had more than an intuitive understanding of the hormonal system and the mutual interactions of the organs. Much of that understanding still escapes us today, even with our lasers, scanners, and other technologies of modern medical research.

In the theory of the Five Evolutive Elements, the kidneys correspond to the north and to cold. The north wind can injure the kidneys, a consideration of great importance in the genesis of chronic illnesses (rheumatic conditions in particular). In traditional medicine, the kidneys correspond to the color black, an association borne out by the unnatural presence of black in the complexion of those suffering from kidney disease. The natural secretion of the kidneys is the saliva that forms at the back of the tongue. The vocal manifestation of the kidneys is the groan or the sigh, the fearful or plaintive voice. The kidneys' psychic manifestation is fear or anxiety. Physiologically, the kidneys' *qi* should rise, but great fear can cause this energy to sink quickly and can result, for example, in loss of control over the sphincter muscles, producing urinary or rectal incontinence in moments of panic.

The psychic entity associated with the kidneys is *zhi*, or determination. One's force of will depends on the well-being of the energies of the kidneys. People who are weak, indecisive, and lacking determination tend to have deficient kidney energy.

One of the functions of kidney *jing* is to produce marrow, which in turn nourishes the bones and ensures the growth and proper development of the skeleton. When the kidneys function properly, in Taoist terms, ossification is healthy, and the fontanels (the membranous intervals in the incompletely ossified cranial bones of the infant) close as they should with age. Deficiencies of the kidneys result in lumbago, fragile bones, defective growth (rickets), and stiff, weak joints, especially those of the knees. People with insufficient kidney *jing* are prone to dental cavities during their early years. Constant dental problems indicate a deficiency of *jing*.

In traditional Chinese medicine, the eyes depend on the liver, although not exclusively: they also depend on the kidneys. Indeed, *jing* expresses itself through the radiance of the pupils. Dilated pupils indicate kidney deficiencies or intoxication. Bags under the eyes denote an insufficiency of kidney *qi* and a problem in the management of body fluids.

As the *Neijing* says, "The *qi* of the kidneys circulates through the ears and when the kidneys are in fullness, the ear can hear the Five Sounds." According to Taoists, ringing in the ears and a diminution of auditory faculties are signs of weak kidney energy.

The central nervous system is nourished by various marrows, and thus by kidney *jing*. Neurological diseases often have their origin in kidney disorders. For example, the neurological problems of senility are attributable to a depletion of *jing;* when there is insufficient *jing*, the marrows cannot be properly nourished. The various problems we associate with old age—loss or loosening of teeth, poor memory, hearing loss and other auditory problems, dizzy spells, and mental confusion—can be traced to the depletion of a person's *jing*.

A Taoist medical text explains that "the kidneys are formed even before the body of the fetus is complete." Taoists consider the kidneys to be the root of life; the weakness or strength of the kidneys is directly related to a person's longevity. Thus, for traditional Chinese medicine, the kidneys are the most important of the human body's vital organs.

The kidneys also manifest themselves in the management of body fluids, in the regulation of breathing, and in processes of excretion. These subjects, however, are well beyond the scope of this work on sexuality, and we will thus not pursue them here.

According to Chinese medicine, hair represents a surplus

of the blood. The blood nourishes the hair, but it is kidney *jing* that hydrates it and gives it vitality and shine. It is therefore possible to assess the general state of the kidneys by the appearance of the hair. Drab, lifeless hair and abnormal hair loss, including premature baldness and alopecia, are signs of possible kidney disorder. The appearance of gray hair, on the other hand, is a sign of the progressive depletion of *jing*, the result of aging. Afflictions of the scalp are therefore treated through interventions aimed at the blood and the kidneys.

THE KIDNEYS GOVERN SEX LIFE

Jing is responsible for procreation, and a deficiency of *jing* can cause sterility. The kidneys' yin *qi*, by producing ancestral energy (*yuanqi*), harnesses the fundamental energy of incarnation known as *chiang*.

In women, the kidneys control the uterus and ensure that conception takes place as it should. The normal functioning of the kidneys also allows a regular menstrual cycle and, together with the liver and the spleen, ensures its proper progression.

Kidney yang (also called the "fire of the *mingmen*" and the "fire of the dragon") governs sexual desire and the libido. An intemperate sex life weakens the kidneys and over the long run will diminish *jing*, the precious treasure of the *xia dantian*.

If a man's kidney and liver energies are normal, his erection—a function that involves the muscles (or, from the Taoist perspective, the sinews)—will also be normal. If there is an insufficiency of either of these two energies, the man will not be able to achieve a complete erection. Kidney yang also controls the sperm barrier, which permits ejaculation at the proper time, in other words, at the moment of orgasm. Weak kidney yang can result in incomplete erections, the inability to have an erection, or a loss of control over the sex act, which can cause premature ejaculation or nocturnal emissions. Young men who masturbate excessively jeopardize their future sexual potential and diminish their *jing* by drawing prematurely on vital reserves. For people in their middle years, too, having sexual relations too frequently and overindulging in alcohol will affect the store of vital potential and invariably diminish precious *jing*. The problem is less worrisome for young men: they can have sexual relations every night (excluding masturbation) without damaging their kidneys, and a good night's sleep will give them sufficient rest to recharge their energy. Additionally, for a young couple, the frequency of their sexual relations will be moderated as a matter of course by the temporary halt occasioned by the woman's period.

In women, an insufficiency of yang fire in the kidneys can be at the origin of a cold energy in the lower abdomen, kidneys, and vagina, and this can cause frigidity and an aversion to sex altogether. Taoists are of the belief that this coldness can be detected by an experienced partner and can somehow be measured by the penis at the moment of penetration.

An insufficiency of kidney yin or of "kidney water" will give rise to frequent and urgent urination, with scanty and concentrated (cloudy or milky) urine.

To bring to a close this broad overview of the physiopathology of the kidneys, an organ that is much more im-

29

portant than Western medicine is inclined to think, we will underscore the interdependent nature of the body's organs, the viscera, or *zang* organs, and the bowels, or *fu* organs. It is essential that they be understood in their interdependence: their functions complement and rely on one another in one grand movement that is both orderly and precise—the cycle of the Five Evolutive Elements. That is how the Chinese of ages past described the general homeostasis of the body. To us this may seem a remarkable achievement for a time when medical technology did not exist. The language is different, but many general theoretical characteristics of ancient practices can be found in modern medicine.

In theory, all the organs—the viscera and the bowels—can influence one another. That is why pathologies tend to be compound and complex, with symptoms that intermingle and intersect with one another to form the symptom complexes (*bian zheng*) with which students of traditional Chinese medicine are familiar.

Without perfect knowledge of this physiopathology (*bian zheng*), the diagnostic basis of traditional Chinese medicine, no lasting, holistic treatment—only symptomatic relief, at best—can take place.

To summarize, from the Taoist perspective the kidneys are the most important organs of the body and must be given particular attention. Sexual excesses and abusing one's sexuality will in general provoke a weakening of kidney *qi*, which manifests itself through feelings of depression and chronic fatigue; lower-back pain (lumbago) and stiffness of the vertebrae; ringing in the ears (tinnitus) and diminished vision; heart palpitations; headaches with dizziness; weakness in the knee joints; and excessive perspiration. These symptoms indicate that the nourishing of the kidneys through the Taoist sexual method needs to begin as soon as possible. The pathologies that are traditionally associated with the kidneys and that have a sexual component will be detailed in the next two chapters.

DETERMINING THE STATE OF THE KIDNEYS' ENERGY BY TAKING THE RADIAL PULSE

Taoists are masters at the art of pulse taking. This art of diagnosing energy disorders is a difficult one; here are the observations of Wang Shuhe, author of *The Pulse Classic*, the standard work on the art of pulse taking, on this subject:

Deficiency of yin is revealed by the absence of the kidney pulse. The following are its signs or symptoms: feelings of heat in the soles of the feet, pains in the hips and the pelvis, loss of *jing* and fatigue.

Yin in excess is indicated by a forceful kidney pulse. Its symptomatic signs are mental confusion, distraction, ringing in the ears.

By applying heavy pressure with the fingers, the kidney pulse is found at the left radial artery close to the bone, about one thumb width above the styloid process, toward the elbow. The strength of the *mingmen* is measured on the other side of the body, on the right radial artery.

In traditional Chinese medicine, taking the pulse at the radial artery is one of the most important of the four steps, or Four Examinations, that constitute the physician's diagnostic inspection of the patient. In China, to say "I'm going to have my pulse taken" is simply another way of saying that one is going to the acupuncturist or herbalist. Pulse taking requires training and experience. The basic treatises on this aspect of Chinese medical diagnostics describe nearly thirty different types of pulses.

The pulse can be taken at different places on the body, and the *Neijing,* alluding to the three traits of the trigram *yijing,* speaks of the pulse of heaven, the pulse of man, and the pulse of the earth. In actual practice, the pulse is taken on each wrist at the radial artery in three different positions. The patient rests his hand on a table, relaxing the muscles of the forearm, while the therapist feels the radial pulse with the fleshy part of his index finger, resting it on the following three pulse points: the "thumb" pulse, located toward the fold of the wrist; the "barrier" pulse, which is felt by pressing on the bony protrusion known as the styloid process; and the "elbow" pulse, located on the other side of the styloid process, toward the elbow. Each position lies one thumb width away from the previous one.

Let us now turn to the relation between the pulse and sexuality. In general, the elbow pulse of both arms represents the energy of the Lower Burner, in other words, the activity of the organs whose functions are believed to center in the area below the navel: the kidneys, urinary bladder, and intestines. But in traditional medicine, the activity of the kidneys is associated with that of the genital organs and the *mingmen,* the Door of Destiny, and the kidneys, related to the element fire, are closely linked to the adrenal glands and original essence (*jing*). Therefore, it is at the elbow that we look for information about a person's sex life.

THE TAO OF LOVE

The pulse can be felt at different levels, or depths: close to the surface, with slight pressure of the finger on the radial artery, or at a deep level, close to the bone. Specialists can feel the pulse at other, intermediate levels.

A classic seventeenth-century work on Chinese pulse theory, *Basic Studies of Acupuncture*, gives the following correlations of pulses with symptom complexes:

Left radial pulse—third (elbow) position (deep)
- Slow pulse (fewer than four beats per respiratory cycle, i.e., one inhalation and one exhalation): In men, this corresponds to thin, clear sperm, weak sexual energy, extreme kidney deficiency, and diarrhea not attributable to other causes. In women, it indicates a "cold uterus"— lack of sexual desire and difficulties in conceiving.
- Minute pulse, deep and intermittent: extreme deficiency of energy. In men, this translates into nonorgasmic involuntary seminal emissions (spermatorrhea) or blood in the urine (hematuria). In women, this kind of pulse is associated with vaginal bleeding and painful periods.
- Very deep pulse: genital sores, inflammation of the delicate genital tissues and membranes.
- Soggy pulse: risk of miscarriage, vaginal blood loss.
- Hidden pulse (the pulse cannot be felt with the finger): absence of sexual energy and desire, heat in the feet (extreme deficiency of yin and yang).

Right radial pulse—third (elbow) position (deep)
- Choppy pulse (the pulse feels rough and bumpy beneath the finger): exhausted sexual energy.
- Long, full, moderate pulse: In men, it is a sign of healthy virility. In women, this pulse is a sign of pregnancy; if

the pulse is "round," it means the child will be a boy; if it is "sharp," the child will be a girl.

- Slow pulse (fewer than four beats per respiratory cycle): the *mingmen* is weak (see above for a discussion of the *mingmen*, or Vital Gate).

NOURISHING THE KIDNEYS FOR A STRONGER SEXUALITY

Taoists think that curbing one's sexual relations is one of the most effective ways to nourish and fortify the kidneys. This approach, however, tends to be more appropriate for monks and ascetics. Fortunately, there are other ways to nourish the kidneys so as to enhance one's sexual capacities. They include toning the kidneys' yin and yang energies and regulating the digestive system through the practice of health exercises (*qigong*), work on the life breath, and diet and herbal therapy.

Kidney-strengthening exercises help to combat the following ailments and symptoms: chronic fatigue subsequent to a protracted illness; loss of vitality and virility; lower-back pains and lumbago; bone disorders of all sorts (decalcification, etc.); ringing in the ears and hearing loss due to factors other than injury; lack of determination; depression and generalized apprehension and anxiety; and kidney and bladder problems.

Yin and yang need to be balanced for new potential to be born; this is true for all living things—plants, animals, and human beings. But most people know the sex act only as something that causes excitation; they have no idea of the many potential dangers that lie hidden behind an act that appears so natural and harmless.

Deaths that occur during sexual intercourse (usually from heart attack or stroke) attest to the strength of the energies that the sex act brings into play. One hears of this kind of occurrence not only in traditional accounts but even today. Ancient legends insist that people who die under such circumstances are transformed into lecherous ghosts, ever in search of sexual union, which, because they are incorporeal, they can never obtain. The risk of coming to such an end actually depends on the health of the kidneys and the cardiovascular system. Excessive use of aphrodisiacs is also believed to increase this risk.

Nourishing the kidneys means working to keep these organs in good shape, even before the first signs of weakness manifest themselves. It is a matter not of taking aphrodisiacs and stimulants but of consuming traditional formulas that belong to the category of tonics. Aphrodisiacs, especially synthetic ones, do nothing but overstimulate such organs as the kidneys, the heart, and the liver and have undesirable side effects that can take forms other than those described above. Toning the kidneys is a long-term effort that involves traditional herbal therapy, proper diet, health exercises (*qigong*), and a healthful lifestyle.

There are certain warning signs that mean the process of toning the kidneys must not be put off any longer. For men these include involuntary seminal emissions, incomplete or limp erections, a noticeable diminishment of libido, and premature ejaculation. For women these signs include lack of sexual feelings during intercourse, feelings of cold in the abdomen and uterus, and absence of vaginal orgasm.

PRACTICING THE TAOIST SEXUAL METHOD

Apart from its ability to nourish the kidneys and preserve the three treasures, the Taoist sexual method offers other benefits: The harmonizing of yin and yang energies during sexual intercourse will improve relations between the two partners on many levels and establish a better equilibrium between them. The restoration of sexual energies nourishes first the kidneys, and then, according to the Taoist theory of the marrows, the brain. The pituitary gland is also stimulated, along with the immune system. The restoration of sexual energy will finally make new strength available for health and intellectual creativity.

A person wishing to preserve kidney energy therefore need not, indeed should not, abstain completely from sexual relations. That course of action is appropriate only for those who take the monastic path. Sexuality needs to be able to express itself both without frustrations and without overpowering passions. Westerners easily accept the first part of this proposition and are more than willing to forgo frustration; only reluctantly, however, do they acknowledge the second part, and, caught in the web of desires, they do not realize that passions can be just as destructive as inhibitions. The Taoist sexual method requires a serene heart, and sexual fantasy is not Taoism's royal road. For any individual, male or female, who is endowed with normal energy, abstaining from sexual relations and indulging in sexual excesses are harmful to vital energy.

THE SEXUAL INTERPLAY OF FIRE AND WATER

The concept of yin-yang has generally been misunderstood in the West. The two terms are often surrounded with mystical meanings or relative value judgments (for example, that yang is better than yin) that they have never had in the East. Yin-yang is a concept, a double adjective that simply denotes changes in the cycles of life in its every possible aspect. Yin-yang also represents a way of thinking that takes into account the two poles of one and the same thing or situation.

Yin-yang theory is perfectly illustrated by the symbol below, representing the profound interaction of yin and yang, which engender each other, stand in opposition to each other, contain part of each other as their own opposites, and follow cyclically one upon the other.

The Chinese character for yang refers to the sunny slope of a hill and has been associated with the qualities of heat, activity, and luminosity. The physical manifestations associated with yang are fever, feelings of heat in the body; organic hyperactivity of various kinds (hypertension, for example); and inflammations and pains of all sorts in the tissues and nerves.

The Chinese character for yin refers to the slope of the hill that remains in the shade year round and is associated with the qualities of cold, passivity, darkness, and interiority and with the following physical manifestations: feelings of cold in various parts of the body; hypoactivity of the organs (organic fatigue); and all ptoses or collapses of the body's tissues (anal ptoses, for example).

38
    There is nothing absolute about this classification of yin and yang, and when these terms are used it is important to specify how they are being used. For example, water is more yin than steam (it is less hot), but it is yang in relation to ice, which is more yin. Moreover, there is always a little yin quality in yang and a little yang quality in yin; one speaks of the yang in yin and the yin in yang, a cycle perfectly described in the *I Ching* (The book of changes) and in the cycle of the four seasons:

Winter is the yin of yin:

Spring is the enclosing of yang within yin:

Summer is the ripening of yang:

Autumn is the first appearance of yin in the heat of summer yang:

The notion of yin-yang involves an intuitive (that is, non-analytic) understanding of subtle Chinese concepts. Consider, for example, the following paradox posited by the philosopher Chouang: "No one lives as long as a child who has died in his earliest years. The centenarian Peng Tseu died before his time. . . ."

Yin and yang create each other; thus in traditional medicine, one says that energy (qi) is born of the blood (yin) and that the blood is driven in its circulatory pathways by energy (yang). If one of the terms is in excess, the other will be stifled and possibly destroyed: for example, in long, serious, chronic diseases, yin—one's essential and hereditary reserves—diminishes considerably, while yang appears strong, manifesting itself in regular, intermittent fevers, dry mouth, intense nervousness, and so on.

For Taoists, the concepts of fire and water are closely connected with the functioning of the kidneys and with sexuality. The right kidney represents fire, while the left kidney is water. Fire governs erection, and water commands ejaculation. Thus, a proper equilibrium between water and fire, between the kidneys' yin and yang, is essential if a harmonious and complete sex life is to be attained. Ancient Chinese texts on sexology frequently compare the sex act to an exchange of energy between the natural elements of fire and water, as we see in the following excerpt:

> The Yellow Emperor said to the Woman of Purity, "I feel tired and anxious. What should I do?" The Woman of Purity answered, "When a woman dominates the man sexually, it is as though a bucket of water was thrown on a candle! The sex life of man and woman can be symbolized by a master cook who

must use the right amount of heat and the right amount of water, no more than is necessary."

The water-fire metaphor has yet another, more graphic meaning: the erect penis is yang-like in its resemblance to a rising flame; the vagina with its secretions is yin-like, filled with fluids. Water and fire also manifest themselves in the physiology of the sex act: the penis swells with heat and retracts in response to cold. When the man is deficient in *mingmen* fire (see above), impotence occurs. When internal secretions are insufficient (deficiency of yin), ejaculation cannot take place. If the woman's uterus is invaded by cold, she becomes frigid. If her internal fluids dry up, her vagina loses its lubrication and inflammations appear.

The task of Taoist alchemy is the preservation of the balance between yin and yang energies, between water and fire; therefore the penis must penetrate the vagina slowly and remain there for some time so that fire can boil water. To this end, Taoists propose different methods for a fruitful sex life; these methods are intended for both men and women and can be classified roughly as follows:

- General advice
- Energy training (*qigong* and *neigong*)
- The use of specific foods or toning formulas
- Massage and moxibustion
- The art of sexual positions
- Work on the heart and the spirit (meditation)

The Taoist master Chen Po Tuan summarized the alchemical work of water and fire in this way: "*Jing* and *shen*, intrinsic vitality and consciousness, are like the joyous embrace of husband and wife."

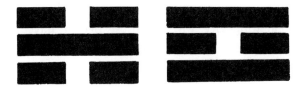

The trigrams of water and fire.

SIGNS OF SEXUAL STRENGTH OR WEAKNESS

The Taoist sexual method offers various ways of gauging a man's or a woman's sexual capacities. Some of these ways are quite useful, others are of purely anecdotal interest. For example, the amount of sperm a young man produces at ejaculation reliably indicates the degree of his sexual vigor: the more sperm, the more *jing*, the proverb says. This statement has led some to think that *jing* and sperm are one and the same thing. According to Taoists, this perspective is too limited.

As we have said, the Chinese Taoists believe that when a man grows old and has sexual relations too often, three symptoms will be observed: lower-back pains, blurry vision, and hearing problems. The ears are thus a good way of checking sexual strength. The Western adage that masturbation causes deafness represents an intuition entirely in line with Taoist teachings. In the *Neijing*, it is also noted that the ears are an emanation of the kidneys; the Taoists have pointed out that most people who enjoy a long life have big ears, and one of the criteria by which they judge the health of the kidneys consists of looking at the shape of the ears. A person with large, fleshy ears, it is said, has plenty of energy and drive, and his sexual energy is strong. On the other hand, people who have small, thin ears rarely enjoy great longevity. Most of these people have weaker, relatively deficient kidneys and thus tend to be passive. One ought not to overgeneralize, however; pulse taking is a better, more serious way of assessing the state of the kidneys than physiognomy.

Other signs that are part of the ancient Taoist science of physiognomy are more anecdotal. Here are a few examples:

SIGN	SIZE OR CHARACTERISTIC	CONCLUSION
Nose and fingers	Small	Short penis
Nose and fingers	Long	Long penis
Lips	Thick	Thick penis
Mouth and fingers	Small	Small, narrow vagina
Lips	Thick	Wide vagina
Lips	Prominent	Supple vagina
Eyes	Sparkling	Well-lubricated vagina
Cheekbones	Prominent	Deep vagina
Wrinkles	Between mouth and nose	Large sexual appetite

In a more serious vein, the ancient Taoists used to consider the angle of a man's erection and his age as ways of determining his sexual vitality. For example, the angle of erection in a thirty-year-old man in good health should be ninety degrees. If his erection is pitched less steeply, his sexual vitality is below normal. Using the following chart, a man can check his own sexual vitality. If the angle of erection is below what it should be for one's age, it is time to practice the sexual Tao.

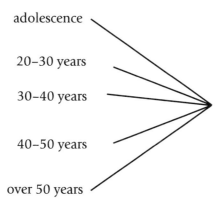

adolescence

20–30 years

30–40 years

40–50 years

over 50 years

The angle of the erection indicates sexual vitality.

SEXUAL FANTASIES AND ILLUSIONS

The Taoist sexual method is concerned above all with preserving the vital forces in such a way that both partners, by developing their bodies, hearts, and minds, can live a long life and enjoy all that our existence here on earth has to offer. This full development of the human potential requires spiritual awareness and a positive outlook. Illusions, fantasies, and sexual avidity are not part of the Taoist program for sexual development. The Taoist master Zuang Tsu was quite clear on this point:

Whoever becomes attached to his fortune will be affronted, whoever attacks power will exhaust himself, whoever lives in idleness will drown in it, whoever revels in the easy life will become its slave: what a sick man's life!

One of the preconditions of longevity is to develop a pure and serene heart. The great Taoist masters of the schools of internal healing summarize the requirements for healthy living in the following way: Preserve original yang *qi* by practicing health exercises. This precious *qi* needs to be stored in the abdominal cinnabar field to fortify the root of life and prevent illness. It is not the work of a single day but requires patience and application. As the proverb says, "How can ten years fit into a single day?" Avoid being trapped by passions that cloud the senses. Passions are actually poisons that dim pure, original thought. The seven emotions are always triggering thoughts that can in turn provoke a kind of anxiety that impedes the circulation of vital energy. A Taoist proverb illustrates this last point: "Those who believe in their dreams sleep all their life."

Eating regular meals and following a proper diet are also necessary, but one must not become obsessed with food or burden the stomach by eating and drinking to excess.

By preserving one's strength and vigor, by cultivating one's consciousness through meditation and emptiness, by taking traditional tonic formulas, a man can attain long life and will not die before his time. But if he does not know the principles of the Taoist sexual method, then paying attention to his diet and his hygiene will be wasted effort. The sexual union of the man and the woman is like the very first creation of the universe. On the other hand, if a man heeds the principles of the sexual act according to the Tao and in harmony with the rules of yin and yang, he will live a joyous life and enjoy the fruits of longevity.

For Taoists, sexuality can be lived in a number of different ways. One is the natural way, that of the Taoists; another is through sexual fantasy, a method even advocated by some psychotherapists. For Taoists, fantasies are a bottomless pit, an illusion with no reality to it whatsoever, a waste of time and energy. Natural sexuality depends on physical, mental, and emotional health, natural biological cycles, the attraction of one partner to the other, and a direct and uncomplicated mutual understanding. If all these conditions are present, then sexuality will be natural and consonant with the way, or Tao, of the universe. If the sex act takes place under these conditions, no energy will be lost and both partners will be spiritually satisfied.

A fantasy-based sex life, however, is totally artificial and verges on unreality. It leads to insatiable hungers and deep feelings of frustration. We can't work out our frustrations by acting out our fantasies. Nor can we be nourished by our illusions, except through self-deception, which always leaves us with a feeling of bitterness or even disgust.

Many newspapers and magazines in the West and some now even in Asia have been promoting the idea of casual sex, which in fact comes with its own norms and codes. This unrealistic point of view is quite the opposite of natural Taoist sexuality, which has no need of fantasy, seduction, the quest for sexual performance, and mutual ego building, all of which are artifices. In short, authentic sexuality has no need for aphrodisiacs, artificial aids, the art of touching, and psychologistic contrivances. A Taoist proverb brings us back to the realities: "Charm and beauty mean very little when they are only external."

THE PRACTICES OF THE SEXUAL TAO

The practices of the male and female sexual Tao aim at balancing the energies in such a way as to foster the natural sexuality advocated by Taoist philosophy. Taoists believe that the great majority of sexual problems stem from organic or energy imbalances and that psychological problems emerge only later from a weak energy base.

The practice of the true sexual Tao amounts simply to a properly oriented lifelong approach to general hygiene, the aim of which is to develop the human being's natural potential. It is in no way a science of aphrodisiacs or a collection of exotic curiosities for the delectation of the Western adventurer who longs for strong sensations.

The methods we present here are traditional ones. They derive from ancient Taoist knowledge of plants, foods, and *qigong* exercises. We describe them in detail, stressing the importance of the nine exercises that together constitute a genuine energy training course of potential benefit to all.

CHAPTER ONE

The Male Sexual Tao

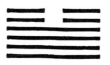

Lack of training and discipline can kill a warrior; lack
of sexual restraint can bring on the permanent sleep
of the hundred bones [death].

—Chinese proverb

WESTERN MEDICINE has a number of categories into
which it classifies male sexual dysfunctions: lack of sexual
desire, impotence (the inability to attain a complete or partial erection), and premature ejaculation, which the Kinsey
Report defines as a man's inability to remain in vaginal
contact with a woman for more than two minutes without
ejaculating.

Western medicine explains male sexual dysfunctions either as psychological in origin—that is, the result of insufficient sexual motivation—or as a circulatory condition, in
which impotence, retarded ejaculation, and premature ejaculation are the products of insufficient vasodilation. For
Taoists, however, as we shall see, sexual dysfunctions are
part of more general processes, what might be called "energy syndromes."

MALE SEXUAL DEFICIENCIES

IMPOTENCE

Impotence is defined in Western medicine as the inability to attain or sustain an erection satisfactory for normal coitus. In Taoist medicine, there are many causes of impotence and many ways of treating it.

When a man cannot attain or sustain an erection, it is usually not for lack of sexual desire. Men who are old and feeble, for example, have sexual desire but cannot satisfy it because their energy is too weak. The inability to attain an erection does not necessarily mean a lack of desire. A Chinese proverb summarizes the situation in this way: "The man's heart is full of desires, but his energy is too undernourished for him to realize them."

Western psychoanalysis would probably respond that the man in this case is suffering from unconscious blocks. Taoists, however, would say that whatever the initial cause—physical, atmospheric, or emotional—an energy deficiency or energy obstruction exists and needs to be addressed.

Taoist medicine distinguishes two categories of impotence: true impotence and energy-related impotence. True impotence means that a man cannot attain erection regardless of external conditions. Energy-related impotence is situational. It depends in large measure on external circumstances and can be the result of psychological blocks or a lack of yang (heat) in the kidneys. In such cases, the penis can become erect but during intercourse will become flaccid again. Some men, for instance, cannot achieve an erection with their spouse but have no such problems with other women.

Taoist medicine attributes impotence to four factors that can disrupt the proper harmony of a man's *qi*: Excessive sexual activity or masturbation during adolescence, which causes a deficiency of *jing* as well as chronic cold in the loins (*mingmen*); psychological shock, which can produce an imbalance between heart energy and kidney energy; liver deficiency and frustration (repressed anger), which can cause a loosening of the sinews in the genital region; an excess of worldly cares (stress) and obsessional thoughts (grief, sadness, melancholy, remorse), which cause an imbalance between the heart and the spleen.

From the standpoint of the energies involved, impotence can be classified into two major categories: that originating in the kidneys and the liver (this type of impotence is treated with tonics for these two organs); and impotence of digestive origin, which is treatable with tonics for the kidneys and the stomach (the stomach-spleen). The herbs that are used to treat kidney-liver impotence can aggravate the second condition, since they can be hard to digest.

PREMATURE EJACULATION

The two-minute threshold that the Kinsey Report uses to define premature ejaculation would strike any Taoist master as much too low, for Taoists believe that ejaculatory control should be total, that the man should be able to ejaculate when he chooses to. The Kinsey definition is all the more inadequate in view of the fact that few women can achieve orgasm in so short a time. Taoist medicine does not adhere to rigid dogma in sexual matters; it prefers to leave people free to find their optimal energy capacities.

It is a further tenet of traditional Chinese medicine that premature ejaculation can lead to impotence if it is left untreated and nothing is done to remedy the energy and emotional factors associated with it.

Premature ejaculation represents, from the standpoint of the energies, an excess of yang in relation to yin. Sperm is yin in relation to sexual desire, which is yang. If yang is overly exuberant, it can no longer contain yin, which escapes prematurely in an involuntary way.

Premature ejaculation is caused by different factors that affect the internal organ's energy balance. These factors include: deficiency of yin (chronic fatigue); deficiency of *qi* (simple fatigue); excess of yang (tension, stress, digestive problems); and disharmony between the heart and the kidneys (as is seen, for example, in certain types of nervous depression). Men suffering from premature ejaculation must be careful to avoid protracted use of kidney yang tonics (see below).

Some women are endowed with a strong libido (yang energy) and weak internal and sexual secretions (deficiency of yin). They have in fact little female energy and consequently tend to weaken the yin of their male partner and provoke premature ejaculation.

MALE SEXUAL FATIGUES

A sexual problem rarely occurs in isolation. It takes form within a specific energy totality, a sort of syndrome or symptom complex. Traditional Chinese medicine recognizes a number of these sexually related syndromes, some of which are described below. Fortunately, a single individual rarely manifests all the symptoms of a given symptom complex. Nonetheless, the presence of a few of these symptoms makes it possible to identify a syndrome, determine its pathological tendencies, and thus avert them.

Deficiency of kidney yin

Signs: Protracted illness, insomnia, night sweats, dry mouth, dry throat, aching in the heels and lumbar region.
Sexual manifestation: Seminal emissions (nocturnal emissions or spermatorrhea).

Deficiency of kidney yang

Signs: Aversion to cold, pallor.
Sexual manifestation: Impotence, seminal emissions.

Deficiency of kidney yin and yang

Signs: Dizziness; ringing in the ears (tinnitus); aching and weakness in the lumbar region and the knee joints; profuse, dilute urine.
Sexual manifestation: Impotence, accompanied by seminal emissions.

Deficiency of *qi* and kidney blood

Signs: Hearing loss, ringing in the ears, dizziness, aching and weakness in the lumbar region and knee joints, frequent nighttime urination.
Sexual manifestation: Seminal emissions and premature ejaculation.

Deficiency of *jing* and kidney *qi*

Signs: Old age or *lao-sun* (fatigue with exhaustion); frequent micturation with pale, dilute urine that becomes more pronounced at night with each urination (sometimes accompanied by urinary incontinence); curvature and softness in the lumbar region and knees.

Sexual manifestation: Seminal emissions, premature ejaculation.

Depletion of kidney *jing*

Signs: Weak constitution, overtiredness, chronic illness, dizziness, ringing in the ears.

Sexual manifestation: Impotence.

Deficiency of spleen and kidney yang

Signs: Cold limbs, pallor, weight loss, mental fatigue, cold and pain in the abdomen, diarrhea with pale stools, early-morning diarrhea, cold and aching in the lower back and knee joints, frequent micturation with dribbling and urgency, frequent nighttime urination, dysuria (difficulties in urinating).

Sexual manifestation: Impotence, seminal emissions.

Deficiency of lung and kidney yin

Signs: Unproductive cough, dry mouth, dry throat, hoarseness, aching and weakness in the lumbar region and knee joints, nervous agitation, disturbed sleep patterns, a feeling of heat emanating from the bones, intermittent fever, night sweats, flushed cheeks.

Sexual manifestation: Exacerbated and unrestrained sexual activity.

TRADITIONAL TAOIST HERBS FOR STRENGTHENING SEXUALITY

The oldest Taoist alchemical texts sometimes refer to the three treasures as the "three herbs," expressing the notion that Taoist alchemy works in ways similar to the actions of natural plants. The ancient Taoists' medical expertise included the use of external elixirs (*wei dan*) derived from plants and sometimes from animal and mineral substances. Here is how the Taoist Wang Che described the action of medicinal herbs: "Medicinal plants are the energy essence of the mountains and rivers, the pure energy of the grasses and the trees. . . . Those who study the Tao must become competent in this subject."

Apart from their medicinal action, Taoist formulas were also used in spiritual exercises, as part of military training, and to strengthen natural vitality. Those used for the latter purpose and for regulating sexuality generally belong to the family of therapeutic agents known as tonics.

Traditional Chinese medicine classifies herbal formulas into eight basic families:

1. Plants that promote sudation (sweating). Plants of this category encourage perspiration and help to eliminate the kind of superficial symptoms that are caused by atmospheric influences (colds, sunstroke, etc.).
2. Plants that promote vomiting. These are the emetic plants that induce vomiting and help rid the body of toxic substances that stagnate in the stomach.
3. Plants that promote purgation. The purgative plants in this category cleanse the digestive system and thus the blood.

4. Plants that encourage the harmonization of the energies. This category includes the harmonizing plants that regularize certain imbalances among two or more vital organs.

5. Plants that induce warming. These plants warm the organs or the energy channels.
6. Plants that induce toning. These plants supplement deficiencies in the organs and the energy channels.
7. Plants that induce purification. These plants rid the energy channels of toxic heat.
8. Plants that induce elimination. These plants eliminate congestions, intestinal stases, or accumulated toxins.

A more recent classification system groups plants and formulas into twenty-one families, as follows:

1. Medicinal plants for fighting superficial symptoms.
2. Medicinal plants for purifying energy of toxic heat, which are useful in treating certain sexual inflammations.
3. Medicinal plants for dispelling wind and removing dampness, which are useful in treating rheumatisms.
4. Medicinal plants for dispelling cold and heat from internal zones, which are useful in treating serious internal cold and for encouraging the circulation of qi in patients of advanced years.
5. Medicinal plants for dispersing dampness.
7. Medicinal plants for inducing vomiting.
8. Medicinal plants for combating constipation.
9. Medicinal plants for stimulating digestion.
10. Medicinal plants for eliminating sputum and mucus.

11. Medicinal plants for regulating energy.
12. Medicinal plants for regulating blood.
13. Medicinal plants for fighting symptoms of congestion and obstruction.

14. Medicinal plants for calming the spirit, which are useful in certain sexual ailments.
15. Medicinal plants for calming the liver and stopping internal wind.
16. Medicinal plants for toning. This family is divided into plants that tone yin, those that tone yang, those that tone blood, and those that tone energy (*qi*).
17. Medicinal plants with an astringent action.
18. Medicinal plants with vermifuge action (i.e., those that eliminate or destroy intestinal worms).
19. Medicinal plants for fighting ulcers and tumors.
20. Medicinal plants for external application.
21. Medicinal plants with antitussive and antiasthmatic action.

In both this system and the earlier one, the most commonly used remedies for sexual deficiencies are found in the category of plants called tonics. This category is further divided into four main subcategories: energy (*qi*) tonics, such as ginseng and astragalus; blood tonics, such as Chinese angelica (*Angelica sinensis*); yin tonics, such as sesame and lily bulb; and yang tonics, such as deer antler.

Certain plants are known for their stimulating effect on male sexuality. Here are some of them, beginning with one that is known the world over.

GINSENG, THE MAJOR TONER OF THE *DANTIAN*

For centuries ginseng has been regarded in the Chinese world as a universal panacea and an aid to longevity. Its ability to balance the circulatory system, stimulate metabolism, and prolong life is widely recognized. Mention of ginseng can be found in the oldest treatises on herbal therapy, including the *Ben Cao* of the "herbalist" emperor Shen Hong, which describes its effects in detail:

> Ginseng fortifies the five vital organs: the liver, the heart, the spleen, the lungs, and the kidneys; it harmonizes yin and yang energies. In other words, it tones energy and blood. Ginseng calms the spirit and dispels fears: it has a sedating effect on the mind (*shen*). Long-term use fortifies the body and prolongs life: this tonic can be used by both men and women.

Ginseng is native to Manchuria, South Korea, and Japan. A number of species are commercially available, including cultivated, semi-wild, and wild varieties; these latter are the best but also the rarest and most costly. The semi-wild roots from China and Korea are quite acceptable alternatives. Probably more has been written about ginseng than about any other plant in existence. A wild thirteen-year-old root will fetch its weight in gold in the shops of Hong Kong.

Ginseng belongs to the family Araliaceae; its scientific name is *Panax schinseng*. Traditional prescriptions usually specify radix ginseng, since it is principally the roots of this plant that are used in medicinal preparations. For over two millennia, the ginseng root has been the most highly regarded tonic plant in the Chinese pharmacopoeia. Here is the classical description of ginseng's tonic properties from the *Ben Cao*:

> The root has a sweet taste and mildly cooling properties. It grows in mountain gorges. It is used to restore the five viscera, harmonize yin and yang, calm the spirit, dispel fears and toxic substances from the body, give brilliance to the eyes, open the vessels of the heart, and bring clarity to the thoughts. Used regularly, it fortifies the body and bestows longevity.

For Taoists, however, these simple definitions are only part of the story: Taoist hermits say that ginseng contains the sap and essence of the earth and the five elements. It develops man's center, his *dantian*, and his spleen. It naturally enhances the three treasures (*san bao*)—*jing, qi,* and *shen*. Ginseng is thus considered a spiritual aid, and many Taoist and Buddhist monks believe it has spiritual effects. Because ginseng increases a person's control over his mind and breathing, many meditators use it regularly as a tonic.

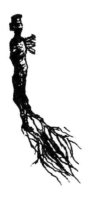

Ginseng.

In the human body, yin represents blood and yang represents energy; accordingly, as modern works on the Chinese pharmacopoeia tell us, ginseng tones energy and blood, which means that this root increases the metabolism and has a measurable effect on the blood corpuscles. That is why ginseng has long been used in China in the treatment of sexual fatigues and deficiencies, lack of appetite, and respiratory problems.

Ginseng can be used by both men and women, and, while in no sense an aphrodisiac, it can help a person maximize his or her sexual energy. Its beneficial, tonic effects are in no way reserved for men. Ginseng does not stimulate the production of male hormones and cause women to grow beards! In fact, in China, herbalists advise ginseng-root preparations for their female patients to alleviate problems associated with menopause.

Herbalists prescribe ginseng to relieve chronic fatigue, whether physical or nervous in origin; stimulate appetite; harmonize menopause; stimulate sexual functions in both men and women; increase virility in older men; and combat senility.

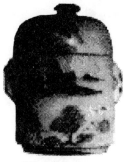

Ginseng Steamer.

Brief summary of the action of ginseng

Botanical reference: Radix ginseng (*Panax schinseng*)

Chinese name: Renshen.

Part used: Dried roots.

Energy: Warm.

Taste: Sweet and slightly bitter.

Dosage: 1 to 9 grams or 60 drops of extract per day.

Actions: Tones energy and blood; calms the mind (*shen*); promotes the production of organic secretions and blood; acts on the spleen, kidney, and lung channels.

Traditional indications: Lack of appetite, chronic fatigue, deficiency of vital energy, sexual fatigue, palpitations, neurasthenia, excessive perspiration, convalescence, anxiety, poor memory, infantile spasms, chronic nausea and vomiting, coughs and chronic respiratory ailments, cardiac problems, kidney, urinary, and uterine ailments, nervous fatigue.

Ginseng should be taken a half hour before meals for treatment of sexual fatigue.

DEER ANTLER OR EXTRACT OF DEER ANTLER

Surely one of the strangest aspects of traditional Chinese medicine, from the Western perspective, is the use of animal products to treat illness and stimulate the body's energies. The Chinese therapeutic arsenal sometimes seems infused with elements of sorcery, making use as it does of such things as gall bladder of bear, lizard skin, and snake blood. Taoists have always been very careful, however, about taking the lives of animals for medical purposes, and many Taoists have been vegetarians.

The animal world can provide hormones and other complex organic substances (tissues, fluids) that are rich in natural energizers, and as long as you are not a vegetarian you can gain much from these age-old remedies, whose effectiveness in recent years has been verified by Soviet scientists who devoted several volumes of research studies to pantocrine, the liquid preparation made from deer antlers.

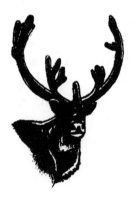

Cornus cervi: *deer antlers may be used medicinally.*

The antlers of young deer (*Cervus nippon*) are removed before they attain a hard, bony consistency and are then prepared as a liquid elixir. This product is now manufactured under state control in both China and parts of the former Soviet Union. The modern preparation is called pantocrine or pantocrin; it is obtained from deer antlers that have been pulverized and then boiled.

Deer antler preparations have been studied for the past fifty years at the Vladivostok Institute of Biological Substances in Siberia. Few Western scientists, however, are truly informed about the results of this research. The first studies, which took place in the Soviet Union well before World

War II, were more concerned with verifying the effects of deer antler extract on the blood than with deepening our biochemical understanding of this substance. In 1969, Dr. Taneyeva of Vladivostok observed a marked increase in muscle tonus. It would be safe to say that scientists in ancient China discovered the hormonal process and, in particular, the important role played by the adrenal glands, as the classic description of deer antler as "the yang root of the kidneys" would seem to indicate. The idea of "root" encompasses such notions as heredity, the parentally transmitted energy that is often referred to in Taoist medical works as "ancestral" energy. And as we now know, the yang root of the kidneys is closely linked to vigorous sexual activity.

Brief summary of the action of deer antler
Scientific name: Cornu cervi pantocrinum, Cervus nippon temminck.
Chinese name: Lou rong.
Part used: Pulverized antler of young deer.
Energy: Warm.
Taste: Sweet and salty.
Actions: Warms the kidneys, fortifies yang, produces sperm, fortifies the blood, stimulates marrow, fortifies bones and the yang root of the kidneys, strengthens male sexual capacity, acts on the liver and kidney channels and the *Chong mai* and *Du mai* channels.
Traditional indications: Weakness and fatigue, male sexual fatigue, intolerance of cold, deficiency of blood, anemia, dizziness, chronic lower-back pain, vaginal hemorrhage caused by weakness, hearing loss attributable to old age, weakness in the limbs and knee joints, impotence, noctur-

nal emissions, leukorrhea, convalescence, chronic illnesses accompanied by sensitivity to cold and asthenia.

ASTRAGALUS ROOT

Chinese experiments have shown that astragalus extends estrus in rats, cures acute nephritis in other animals, promotes diuresis, and combats certain types of bacteria. Astragalus preparations are frequently used in cases of suppuration (pus formation): astragalus brings pustules to a head and aids in their healing. It has a beneficial effect in cases of gangrene and noncancerous tumors. It is a yang-type sexual tonic that bestows energy and prolongs virility.

Found in herbal formulas of all sorts, astragalus tones and enhances synergistic effects; for this reason people with hypertension or what used to be known as sanguine constitutions should avoid using it. Its tonic action, like that of ginseng, makes it an effective treatment for hemorrhoids and fistulas.

Brief summary of the action of astragalus
Botanical reference: Astragalus membranaceus, A. mongholicus, A. hoantschy
Chinese name: Huang qi.
Energy: Neutral.
Taste: Sweet.
Actions: Tones all body functions, strengthens defenses, clears pus, stops abnormal sweating, works as a sexual tonic.
Properties: Stimulant, diuretic, tonic, healant, antiseptic.
Energy profile: Astragalus root is an important remedy in the

traditional Chinese phamacopoeia; it is available from certain Chinese grocery stores as dried roots or from Chinese herbalist pharmacies as astragalus extract. Less costly than the more widely known ginseng, this tonic plant stimulates yang energy. It is therefore recommended for the kidneys, lungs, energy, and blood. A powerful sexual tonic, it is used in combination with ginseng to help concentrate the sperm and increase its density.

Traditional indications: Fatigue, intolerance of cold, sweating with asthenia, loose stools or diarrhea, tendency to infection, pimples.

Use and preparation: Decoction of astragalus root can be prepared according to the following method, which Chinese therapists use. Place ten grams of *huang qi* root in an enamel pot. Add two cups of water and bring to a boil over a low flame. Continue boiling until the liquid is reduced by half. Strain. The decoction should be drunk hot in two doses: the first in the morning on waking, and the second before the noonday meal. This cure should be continued for two to three weeks and repeated if necessary. Do not begin this treatment if you have influenzal fever; if you have already begun the cure and then develop influenzal fever, you should discontinue it.

It is important to consider a plant's nature and energy before deciding whether or not to use it. Ginseng and astragalus are energy tonics and are effective for treating depletion of sexual energy in men (and in some cases in women). But whereas ginseng decreases micturation (urination), astragalus promotes it. A person suffering from edema would therefore do better to use astragalus root rather than ginseng.

Other Plants with Sexually Related Actions

PLANT	EFFECT ON SEXUAL ENERGIES
Cassia tora	Tones yin
Rehmannia glutinosa	Tones yin
Cornus officinalis	Astringent, retains substances, tones and warms kidney yang
Water plantain	Dispels humidity
Poria cocos	Dispels humidity
Peony	Warms blood
Monkey prostate (animal substance)	Tones yang
Deer antler extract	Tones jing and marrows
Cinnamomum cassia	Tones and warms kidney yang
Dioscorea opposita	Tones and warms kidney yang
Lycium sinensis	Nourishes blood, liver, and kidney yin
Eucommia ulminoides	Warms and tones the liver and kidneys, strengthens the bones, sinews, and muscles
Angelica sinensis	Nourishes and mobilizes blood by toning blood of the liver

CLASSIC TAOIST FORMULAS FOR STRENGTHENING MALE SEXUALITY

Sexual problems are generally treated with classical formulas, some of which are found in the earliest traditional medical treatises, such as the *Shang Han Lun* (The treatise on febrile diseases). These formulas use plants from the following categories:

- Energy tonics and blood tonics, used in combination to strengthen both energy and blood.
- Yin tonics and yang tonics, used in combination to strengthen yin-yang balance.

- Yin tonics, for toning the kidneys in cases of kidney yin deficiency.
- Yang tonics, for treating deficiencies of kidney yang.
- Energy tonics, to treat deficiencies of spleen and digestive weaknesses.
- Blood tonics, for treating mental and psychological disorders.

Listed below are the traditional medicinal formulas that are most appropriate for treating male sexual problems. Their composition is precise, and they are usually prepared by specialized herbalists as either decoctions or soluble powders. Follow the herbalist's instructions as to the proper dose.

Kidney-toning pill for men

Nan Xing Bu Shen Wan

Composition: Rehmannia glutinosa, Aconite carmichaeli, Cornus officinalis (Shan Zhu Yu), *Alisma orientale* (Xe Xie), *Plantago asiatica* (Che Qian Zi), *Cinnamomum cassia* (Rou Gui).

Actions: Tones and warms kidney yang, Tones kidney *qi* and kidney *jing*, diuretic.

General indications: Depletion of kidney yang, *qi*, and *jing*; lower-back pain; urinary incontinence; frequent, scanty urination, dribbling; cold extremities.

Sexual indications: Sexual asthenia.

Format and dosage: Gel capsules, twenty per box (Lanzhou Fo Ci Pharmaceutical Factory; Lanzhou Gansu). One capsule twice daily, morning and evening.

Pill for the right kidney

You Gui Wan

Composition: Colla colmu cervi cortex, *Cinnamomum cassia* (Rou Gui), *Cornus officinalis* (Shan Zhu Yu), *Lycium sinensis*

(Gou Qi Zi), *Eucommia ulminoides* (Du Zhong), *Aconite carmichaeli*, *Rehmannia praeparata* (Shou Di Huang), semen *Cuscuta sinensis*, *Angelica sinensis* (Dang Gui).

Actions: Nourishes and mobilizes blood by toning the blood of the liver, tones and warms kidney yang, nourishes blood, tones *jing*.

General indications: Depletion of kidney yang with weakness of *yuanqi*, chronic nephritis, edema in the lower extremities, diabetes, exhaustion following protracted illness, intolerance of cold, aching and weakness in the lumbar region and knee joints, loose stools, occasionally lienteric (containing undigested food), urinary incontinence.

Sexual indications: Impotence, spermatorrhea, sterility.

Format and administration: This medicine is taken in the form of boluses, that is, traditional Chinese pills containing pulverized herbs bound together with honey. To make the boluses, reduce the ingredients to a powder, add a little honey, and roll into balls the size of green peas. Take six to twelve grams, two or three times a day, with a little warm water.

Decoction: Fifty to eighty grams per liter. Reduce to forty centiliters to be taken over the course of a day in three or four doses.

Drink for the right kidney

You Gui Yin

Composition: Rehmannia praeparata (Shou Di Huang), *Cinnamomum cassia* (Rou Gui), *Lycium sinensis* (Gou Qi Zi), *Eucommia ulminoides* (Du Zhong), *Aconite carmichaeli*, *Cornus officinalis* (Shan Zhu Yu), *Glycyrrhiza uralensis* (Gan Cao).

Actions: Tones and warms kidney yang, tones *jing.*

General indications: Depletion of kidney yang; true cold with pseudo-heat symptoms caused by a preponderance of yin with upward floating of deficient yang; diabetes insipidus; chronic nephritis; chronic bronchitis; cold extremities; aversion to cold; aching and weakness in the lumbar region and knee joints; abdominal pain; loose stools; frequent urination, with profuse and dilute urine; urinary incontinence.

Sexual indications: Impotence, spermatorrhea, premature ejaculation.

Format and administration: As a decoction, fifty to sixty grams per liter. Reduce to forty centiliters to be taken over the course of a day in three or four doses.

Kidney-toning pill for men

Nan Xing Bu Shen Wan

Composition: Rehmannia praeparata (Shou Di Huang), *Poria cocos* (Fu Ling), *Paeonia alba* (Bai Shao Yao), *Schisandra sinensis* (Wu Wei Zi), *Aconite carmichaeli, Cornus officinalis* (Shan Zhu Yu), *Alisma orientale* (Xe Xie), *Plantago asiatica* (Che Qian Zi), *Cinnamomum cassia* (Rou Gui).

Actions: Tones and warms kidney yang, tones kidney *qi* and kidney *jing,* acts as a diuretic.

General indications: Depletion of kidney yang, *qi,* and *jing;* lower-back pain; urinary incontinence; frequent, scanty urination and dribbling; cold extremities.

Sexual indications: Sexual asthenia.

Format and administration: Gel capsules, twenty per box (Lanzhou Fo Ci Pharmaceutical Factory; Lanzhou Gansu). One capsule twice daily, morning and evening.

Fertility-promoting pill

Zan Yu Dan

Composition: Aconite carmichaeli, Herba Cistanchis desedicolae, *Epimedium grandiflora* (Yin Yang Huo), *Allium sativum* (Da Suan), *Cornus officinalis* (Shan Zhu Yu), *Rehmannia praeparata* (Shou Di Huang), *Lycium sinensis* (Gou Qi Zi), *Cinnamomum cassia* (Rou Gui), *Morinda officinalis* (Ba Ji Tian), fructus *Cnidii Monnieri*, Rh *Curculiginis orchioidis*, *Eucommia ulminoides* (Du Zhong), *Angelica sinensis* (Dang Gui), *Atractylodes macrocephala* (Bai Zhu).

Actions: Tones and warms the kidneys.

General indications: Depletion of kidney yang (insufficiency of *mingmen* fire) and of *yuanqi*, apathy, lack of determination, lumbago, weakness in the lumbar area, pallor.

Sexual indications: Infertility, impotence.

Format and administration: For boluses, reduce the ingredients to a powder, then add a little honey and form pills the size of green peas. Take three to six grams a day in two to three doses with a little hot water. In decoction, sixty to one hundred grams per liter. Reduce to forty centiliters to be taken over the course of a day in three to four doses.

Lower-back-fortifying and kidney-strengthening tablet

Yao Jian Shen Pian

Composition: Rhizoma *Cibotii barometz*, *Eucommia ulminoides* (Du Zhong), *Loranthus parasiticus* (Sang Ji Sheng), *Poria cocos* (Fu Ling), caulis *Millettiae reticulatae*, fructus *Rosae*, *Laevigatate sclerotium*, *Cordyceps sinensis*, fructus *Rubi chingii*.

Actions: Tones kidney *qi* and yang, strengthens the sinews and bones.

General indications: Depletion of kidney yang (often the result of sexual intemperance in men); chronic nephritis; lumbago; weakness in the lumbar region, waist, and knee joints; lower-back pain; vertigo; tinnitus; frequent, scanty urination, with dribbling; dyspnea; poor memory; fatigue.

Sexual indications: Fatigue following sexual excesses.

Format and administration: Pills, in bottles of one hundred (United Pharmaceutical Manufactory, Guangzhou, Guangdong). Four pills, once or twice a day, with a little warm water.

Kidney-toning cistanche pill

Cong Rong Bu Shen Wan

Composition: Cistanchis desenicolae, semen *Cuscuta sinensis, Rehmannia praeparata* (Shou Di Huang), *Schisandra sinensis* (Wu Wei Zi).

Actions: Nourishes yin and tones kidney *jing* and yang, strengthens sinews and bones.

General indications: Depletion of kidney yin, yang, and *jing;* lumbago; weakness in the lumbar area and knees; constipation in elderly patients; diminished vision; frequent urination; profuse perspiration.

Sexual indications: Impotence, premature ejaculation, spermatorrhea.

Format and administration: Pills, in bottles of two hundred (Lanzhou Fo Ci Pharmaceutical Factory; Lanzhou). Eight pills, three times a day, with a little warm water.

The next four formulas are traditional Taoist liquors that are used to strengthen sexual energies; they are prepared by decocting the ingredients in rice wine or other strong alcohol. The resulting liquor is then stored in a dark place for two to three months.

Golden phoenix liquor

Ingredients: Rehmannia praeparata (Shou Di Huang), *Rehmannia glutinosa* (Sheng Di Huang), *Angelica sinensis* (Dang Gui), *Ophiopogon japonicus* (Mai Men Dong), *Lycium sinensis* (Gou Qi Zi), *Epimedium grandiflora* (Yin Yang Huo), *Amomum villosum*.

Steep all the ingredients together in rice wine for at least a month.

Actions: Tones kidney yin and yang, supplements *jing* and the energy of the *dantian*.

General indications: Chronic fatigue.

Sexual indications: Sexual asthenia.

Wine of the two immortals

Ingredients: Cornu cervi (Lu Rong), *Cervus Nippon* jelly, *Chinemys reevesii*, *Chinemys reevesii* jelly, *Lycium sinensis* (Gou Qi Zi), *Panax schinseng* (Ren Shen), *Angelica sinensis* (Dang Gui), *Astragalus membraneceus*.

Steep all ingredients together in rice wine for at least three months.

Actions: Nourishes yin and marrow, tones and supplements *qi* of the *dantian*, tones the kidneys, enhances the three treasures.

General indications: Lower-back pain.

Sexual indications: Seminal emissions.

Li Shih-chen's aphrodisiac formula

Li Shih-chen is China's most renowned herbalist; his magisterial work, *Pen-ts'ao Kang-mu* (Compendium of materia medica), contains thousands of medicinal formulas, including this ancient Taoist "aphrodisiac pill."

Ingredients: Cyperus rotundus (Xiang Fu), *Poria cocos* (Fu Ling mushroom), and honey, as a binder for the other two in-gredients.

Actions: Tones *jing* and yang *qi*.

Sexual indications: Sexual fatigue, impotence, lack of sexual desire.

Dosage: One to three boluses for fifteen days.

Virile wine

Ingredients: Dioscorea opposita (10 grams), *Cornus officinalis* (10 grams), *Schisandra sinensis* (10 grams), *Panax schinseng* (10 grams).

Actions: Tones *jing,* yang *qi,* the spleen, the stomach, mus-cles, and tendons.

Sexual indications: Sexual fatigue, impotence.

This Taoist wine, a major tonic with both sexual and di-gestive properties, is prepared by placing the ingredients in a liter of strong alcohol and letting them steep for at least two months.

Administration: One to two glasses a day. (Do not begin this treatment in midsummer.)

COMMERCIALLY MANUFACTURED FORMULAS FOR MALE SEXUALITY

Pills of commercial manufacture can be either classic for-mulas or a single herb prepared for mass-market consump-tion. The following are formulas with sexual actions.

Gecko Major Supplementation Pills
Ge Jie Da Bu Wan

Actions: Tones bones, lungs, kidneys, and liver; strengthens the heart; fortifies, relaxes, and calms the spleen, stomach, bones, and sinews; calms rebellious *qi*.

General indications: Asthma, fatigue, aching bones, dizziness, lumbago, nightmares, anxiety, tinnitus, frequent urination, incipient osteoporosis, coughing, deficiencies of the lungs and kidneys.

Sexual indications: Sexual exhaustion, impotence.

Recommended dosage: Three to five pills, taken after breakfast.

Rehmannia Six Pills

Liu Wei Di Huang Wan

Actions: Nourishes kidney yin, supplements yin, tones blood, calms the heart, calms the emotions, stabilizes *shen*, tones kidney yin and yang.

General indications: Fatigue, weakness in the knee joints, dizziness, nervousness, hypertension, senility, tinnitus, spermatorrhea, hematuria, deficiencies of blood and yin, constipation, diabetes, sore throat, excessive thirst.

Sexual indications: Sexual fatigue, impotence resulting from illness.

Recommended dosage: Eight to sixteen pills, three times a day. Appropriate for both men and women.

Ginseng Extract

Panax schinseng extractum

Actions: Tones *qi* and *yuanqi*; nourishes body fluid; calms *shen*; tones the lungs; develops the center and earth (one of the five elements); nourishes the three treasures, *jing, qi,* and *shen*; stimulates perceptions; and facilitates meditation.

General indications: Neurasthenia, fatigue, loss of appetite, indigestion, headaches, insomnia, poor memory, abdominal pains, dysentery, shock, chronic fever, deficiency of lung and heart *qi*.

Sexual indications: Sexual fatigue, impotence.

Recommended dosage: Sixty drops, two or three times a day.
Recommended for all types of constitutions.

Deer Antler Extract

Pantocrine

Actions: Tones the kidneys, liver, heart, and brain; stimulates blood circulation; tones marrow and yang; promotes longevity; enhances physical form and vitality.

General indications: Neurasthenia following a heart attack, poor memory, hair loss.

Sexual indications: Sexual fatigue, impotence.

Recommended dosage: Sixty drops, twice a day.

Polygonatum "Black-Head" Pill

Shou Wu Pian

Actions: Tones the liver and kidneys, supplements *jing* and blood, detoxifies and tones blood, tones the muscles and bones, supplements sperm and stimulates fertility, promotes longevity, develops the element wood.

General indications: Liver and kidney deficiencies, constipation, skin ailments, premature graying of hair, weakness in the lumbar region and the knees, chronic leukorrhea, flatulence, intestinal difficulties.

Sexual indications: Sexual fatigue, premature ejaculation.

Recommended dosage: Five pills, three times a day.

Heart-Supplementing and Spirit-Quieting Pill

Tian Wang Pu Xin Tan

Actions: Nourishes the tired heart, calms emotional instability.

General indications: Lassitude, anxiety, tinnitus, palpitations, breathing difficulties, imsomnia, poor memory, night sweats.

Sexual indications: Sexual difficulties due to anxiety, premature ejaculation, sexual debilitation.

Recommended dosage: Five pills, three times a day.

Tiger Bone Pill

Tu Ku Wan

Actions: Fortifies the bones and sinews, reduces spasms, relaxes the muscles, stimulates blood circulation.

General indications: Flatulence, rheumatic pains *(bi)*, lumbago, gout, swelling of the limbs, arthritis, infantile spasms, shaking.

Sexual indications: Treats impotence resulting from weakness of the tendons and the muscles.

Recommended dosage: Four to eight pills, morning and night.

Three Treasures Pill

Tzepao San Pien Pills

Actions: Tones *jing*, tones the brain, works as a major sexual tonic.

General indications: Weakness, senility, impotence, neurasthenia, kidney ailments, dizziness, poor memory, pimples on the back and chest, excessive perspiration, pallor, insomnia.

Sexual indications: Sexual fatigue, impotence.

Recommended dosage: One pill, once a day. Also available in vials; drink one-third to one vial a day.

NOURISHING SEXUALITY THROUGH DIET

Taoist culture recognizes the utility of certain foods for the maintenance of good health. Some of these belong to the category of tonics. These foods, as one might expect, stimulate the sexual functions.

In the *Neijing*, the physician Qi Bo addresses the Yellow Emperor as follows:

> In ancient times some men knew the Tao. They followed the rules of yin and yang; they could control their emotions and knew how to avoid eating and drinking too little or too much by taking into account the five celestial movements, the five terrestrial tastes, and the four seasons.

Chinese medicine classifies therapeutic foods in much the same way it classifies medicinal plants: there are foods for superficial symptoms, for dispelling heat, for toning, and so on. Here are some foods that are recognized for their sexual properties. They are particularly useful in cases of sexual fatigue and impotence:

FOOD	ENERGY ACTION
Longan, black carp, potato, red grape, chicken, Lung yen, grapes, wine, Chinese dates	*Qi* tonics
Nuts, grapes and old wine, litchis	Blood tonics
Litchis, nuts, grapes	Kidney tonics
Dried ginger, seaweed, sea cucumber	Yang tonics
Chicken, lamb, beef, kidneys, particularly kidney bouillon	*Jing* tonics (foods that restore sexual energy)
Egg yolks, duck eggs, pork, squid, and many others	Yin tonics

Note that animal products figure prominently among foods in this category. Respectful of the world of nature, particularly of its living creatures, Taoists are often repelled by the idea of eating meat; these foods thus constitute an exception in the Taoist tradition and are to be used on an exceptional basis. Taoists have tended to be vegetarians out of respect for animal life in all its forms. Some tonic dishes do, however, make use of meats and fish, and Taoists have always attached a great deal of importance to the observation that human organs can be treated with the corresponding organs of animals: for example, animal liver for toning the human liver, animal kidneys for fortifying the human kidneys, and so on.

SIMPLIFIED DIETARY RECOMMENDATIONS FOR SEXUAL DEFICIENCIES

In China certain conditions *(sho)* are considered the warning signs of organ or energy deficiencies that can lead to impotence or disease. As noted earlier, traditional Chinese medicine groups these signs into symptom complexes that indicate the particular pathological area that needs to be remedied. Sexual excesses can lead to these major fatigues, as well as to other fatigues and ailments.

Here are some of the principal deficiency conditions that can manifest themselves in the diminishment of sexual capacities. These energy syndromes take up from those developed earlier in a more simplified way in the section on sexual problems:

Deficient Vital Gate (Shen Men)

Indications: Pallor, joint pains, weakness in the legs, neurasthenia, ejaculation with thin sperm, along with feelings of cold and a thready pulse.

Traditional Taoist dietary recommendation: Foods that warm kidney yang, such as black sesame seeds, chicken livers (or livers of other fowl), kidneys, hazelnuts, strawberry and raspberry compote.

Emotional troubles affecting the spleen and the heart

Indications: Dull or yellow complexion, lack of appetite, fatigue, depression.

Traditional Taoist dietary recommendation: Red dates, decoction of dates, beef, two cups of coffee per week.

Kidney-damaging fear

Indications: Suspicion, fear, lack of courage, palpitations, insomnia.

Traditional Taoist dietary recommendation: Fortify the kidneys and calm the spirit with a diet of millet, mulberries, wheat (flakes or berries), hops, decoctions of thyme, rosemary, lily flowers, ginseng.

Deficient yin and pseudo-excess of yang

Indications: Great sexual desire; very premature ejaculation; insomnia due to excessive ideation; dry throat; vision difficulties; concentrated urine, dark yellow or orange in color; rapid, thready pulse; red tongue.

Traditional Taoist dietary recommendation: Pear peelings, asparagus, coconut milk, duck, chicken eggs, mulberries, raw oysters, pork.

Deficient energy in the Middle Burner

Indications: Inability to maintain a firm erection; short-windedness; weakness; lack of appetite; deep, thready pulse; thin, moist coating on the tongue.

Traditional Taoist dietary recommendation: Eggs of the swallow, beef, pheasant, hare, short-grain rice, sweet white rice, brown sugar, cherries, chicken, coconut, red dates, dates, olive oil.

Deficient kidney yang energy

Indications: Complete inability to attain erection, aching joints, weakness in the legs, seminal emissions, premature ejaculation, coldness in the limbs.

Traditional Taoist dietary recommendation: The same as for deficient Vital Gate.

Congested liver energy

Indications: Pain in the sides, frequent eructation (belching).

Traditional Taoist dietary recommendation: Disperse the energy of the liver channel with a decoction of orange peels and leaves and flowers of the mandarin orange.

Kidney-damaging sexual excesses

Indications: Coughing, vomiting, lumbago, weakness in the knees, coldness in the limbs, seminal emissions and premature ejaculation, hot flushes throughout the body.

Traditional Taoist dietary recommendation: Black sesame seeds, black sesame oil (available from Chinese grocery stores), beef marrow, perch, strawberry and raspberry compote, hazelnuts (soaked in water overnight).

Naturally, with each of these energy disorders, not all the symptoms will appear at the same time. The recommended foods should be eaten at least two times a week, with meals.

SIMPLE RECIPES FOR MALE SEXUALITY

Here are a few Taoist recipes for supplementing and improving the sexual energies. They are based on the energy principles of food and on the interplay of the five flavors.

Rice with cistanche

Indications: Impotence, infertility, constipation, sensitivity to cold.

Counter-indications: Signs of heat, fever.

Ingredients: 100 grams white rice; 30 grams saline (herba cistanchis); 10 grams lean mutton, cut into small pieces; 10 milliliters rice wine; 10 grams fresh ginger root; 10 grams chives; 5 grams salt.

Actions: Cistanche tones the kidneys and helps add water bulk to the large intestine.

Preparation: Cut the ginger in slices. Wrap in a piece of cheesecloth along with the cistanche and tie the ends. Let soak in 700 milliliters of water for 1 hour. Boil for 20 minutes, then remove the packet. Add the rice, the mutton, and the rice wine to the liquid that remains. Boil over a low flame for 20 minutes. Add the chives and the salt. Cook for 3 more minutes.

Eat this dish twice a week for a month.

Cornmeal and chicken soup for increasing sexual energy

Ingredients: Two chicken wings, chopped fine; one beaten egg; 5 tablespoons cornmeal; 3 cups water; ¼ cup margarine or sesame oil; 1 teaspoon sea salt; 1 tablespoon cow or goat milk.

Preparation: Combine the water, margarine, salt, and cornmeal. Bring to a boil. Add the chopped chicken wings and return to a boil while stirring well.

Actions: This excellent *qi* tonic also tones the sexual functions and fortifies the heart.

Kidney bouillon for toning the kidneys

Ingredients: Pork kidneys, salt, and the herbs Du Zhong (radix *Eucommiae*) and He Shou Wu (radix *Polygoni multiflori*).

Preparation: Cover two pork kidneys with salt for 24 hours. The next day, rinse the kidneys and blanch in boiling water. In a separate pot, boil the herbs (10 grams of each) in 2 cups of water for an hour, covered and over a low flame. Strain, discard the herbs, and return the remaining liquid (there should be about 1 cup) to the pot. Rinse the kidneys once again and add to the liquid from the herbs; cook for another half hour. Drink the broth. You can also eat the kidneys themselves, if you like, but the tonic properties will be mostly in the broth.

Actions: According to Taoists, this preparation enters the liver and kidney channels and fortifies the sinews, bones, kidneys, and sexual functions in general. It is a tonic and can be used occasionally to vitalize the body and promote longevity. The herb Du Zhong is named after a Taoist hermit who is reputed to have attained enlightenment after eating some of it. This preparation is believed beneficial to both the body and the spirit.

Gray shrimp sauté

Indications: Impotence, weakness in the legs and lumbar area.

Counter-indications: Signs of heat, facial flushing, fear of perspiration, thirst.

Ingredients: 50 grams Chinese leeks, 50 grams gray shrimps, 10 milliliters rice wine, 10 grams ginger, 10 grams chives, rapeseed oil.

Leek soup

Actions: Excellent for toning *qi* and the sexual functions. Only the white part of the leek should be eaten. It is an excellent remedy for premature ejaculation.

Preparation: In a liter of water, simmer 50 grams of the white part of the leek over a low flame for 1 to 2 hours.

EXERCISES FOR INCREASING SEXUAL STRENGTH

Generally speaking, there are two ways to increase sexual strength: diet (which should be understood as including both therapeutic plants and toning foods) and physical discipline. While diet may be the simpler of the two methods, it is also the one on which a person can become the most dependent.

The ancient Taoists invented a number of exercises whose purpose was to help develop effective physical and mental strength for daily life and to remedy bodily deficiencies that might hinder a person from embarking on spiritual practices. Some of these methods are specifically designed to tone sexual strength and constitute a genuine and total therapy for the individual who seeks to take control of his energy economy. The exercises and techniques given below are designed to develop the sexual energies. Drawn from the esoteric traditions of *daoyin*, *qigong*, and *neigong*, they work for the most part by toning the kidney or toning *jing*.

Mounted archer's pose for strengthening the kidneys

This exercise is a stationary pose; its toning action strengthens the kidneys. It is one of the best known of all Chinese health exercises, having been adopted by many martial arts schools in China and Japan. Also called the horseman's pose, it figures in many of the ancient medical classics. Here are some of the benefits it confers:

- Fortifies the kidneys (in the broad sense of the term, as explained above).
- Stimulates circulation of blood and improves the quality of blood.
- Calms mental overexcitement and strengthens courage in the face of the challenges of daily life.
- Stimulates the spleen and the stomach and fortifies digestion.

Spread your legs so that they are slightly more than shoulder-width apart.

Without lifting your heels from the floor, bend your knees, as though you were riding a horse. Cross your arms in front of your chest.

Then pull one of your arms back, as though you were drawing back a bowstring.

Return to the starting, crossed-armed position; as you do this, inhale.

Repeat this sequence at least seven times.

This exercise provides a good foundation on which to begin the practice of *qigong* for strengthening male sexuality.

Daoyin for strengthening the kidneys and sexuality

Sit cross-legged on the floor. Cover your ears with your hands in such a way that your fingers are behind your head. Raise your elbows to the sides.

Keeping your hips facing forward, rotate your torso to the left as you exhale gently.

Bring your torso back to the starting position; as you do this, inhale. Now do the same thing again, but this time to the right.

Repeat this sequence fifteen times.

Breathe naturally as you perform these movements. Both your breathing and the movements should be unforced.

After you have performed this sequence fifteen times, massage each arm in an upward direction from the forearm to the upper arm. Massage the inside of your arm first, then the outside. Do this fifteen times.

This exercise increases resistance to disease, strengthens vitality and courage, and combats kidney and bladder troubles of all sorts. It gently stimulates and strengthens the sexual energies.

Neigong kidney massage

The loins protect the kidneys; they are a refuge for *jing*, and thus ensure reproduction. The lumbar vertebrae are a major intersection of the body's energies. Massaging this area with gentle taps tones the kidneys, increases energy, and drains the channels.

Here is how one Taoist internal-exercise text explains the procedure:

> Rub your hands together to produce heat; inhale cool *qi* through the nose, then exhale it slowly, still through the nose; then massage the loins with your hands, which you have first warmed by rubbing them together. Then rub your hands together again and massage your kidneys ninety times with both hands. This exercise strengthens yang energy, relieves lower-back pains, and increases urinary excretions.

Cinnabar field massage

This method consists of massaging the cinnabar field, or *dantian*, which Taoists call the Elixir Field or Vital Gate. The abdomen protects the *dantian*, the storehouse for vital energy in men, the site of the uterus in women. This area plays an important role as a reservoir for sexual energies. The ancient Taoists referred to this method as the *dantian*, or Vital Gate, massage.

Massaging this area tones kidney energy, fortifies the spleen and stomach, promotes the circulation of vital energy in the channels, and improves digestion. This massage also mobilizes energy, making it immediately available.

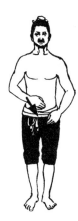 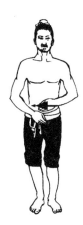

Cinnabar field massage.

Press with your fingers or the palm of your hand against the center of your lower abdomen, then rotate; be sure to keep the movement circular. Your hand should always be in contact with the skin but not pull too strongly against it. Massage your cinnabar field in this way thirty-six times. As you do this, check to see if your penis has risen slightly, which will indicate that the pressure is reaching the genital area. This exercise takes several minutes. You should stop when you feel a sensation of heat in your lower abdomen.

This technique, if practiced regularly, increases sexual energy and can remedy impotence. Its effectiveness has led many modern physicians to attempt to explain it in terms of Western medical science. According to these physicians, this massage stimulates the prostate, which activates the sperm. It is not surprising, therefore, that the cinnabar field massage can also increase fertility.

Foot massage for fortifying *jing* and the sexual organs

The feet are not only useful instruments for getting us from one place to another, they are also an indicator of the state of health of the entire body. Chinese physicians since time immemorial have paid particular attention to the feet and have developed effective methods to fortify health by treating the feet. Foot massage is one of the simplest and most easily practiced of these methods.

The most important massage point on the sole of the foot is called the *yongquan* point (literally, the boiling spring); it is located at the center of the arch, on the kidney channel (this channel goes from the little toe through the arch of the foot, the ankle, leg, spinal column, abdomen, chest, and throat, all the way to the base of the tongue).

The second most important point on the sole of the foot is the heel; this point corresponds to the sexual organs.

Frequent massage of the *yongquan* point is an effective way to unblock the kidney channel, regularize energy, and activate the circulation of blood. The body is invigorated by the flow of vital energy, kidney functions improve, the sexual organs are toned, the immune system is strengthened, and the entire organism is better able to resist the wear and tear of daily life.

A well-known Chinese therapist, Chen Zhi, used to prescribe the following foot massage. Here is the procedure as he described it:

The *yongquan* point is found on the arch of the foot, where dampness enters. Every day, massage this point on each foot—first one foot, then the other—with the thumb of your hand as you hold your toes with the other hand. After a little while, when you feel the heat spread across the entire sole of your foot, wiggle your toes gently.

Grasping the toes of your foot with one hand, massage the *yongquan* point with the thumb of your other hand thirty-six times without stopping. Try to keep a fairly exact count.

Perform this massage gently until the sole of the foot becomes quite warm. You can enhance this effect by increasing the pressure you exert with your thumb on the *yongquan* point.

If you perform this exercise regularly, you will definitely notice not only its overall health benefits but also its positive effects on your sexual health.

Urinating on tiptoes

Urinating while standing on tiptoes fortifies the kidneys by stimulating the *yongquan* point and increases control of the flow of urine. This Taoist exercise is also a cure for impotence and premature ejaculation. A simple exercise to perform, it should be done with your back straight and your teeth clenched, which will help produce a forceful urine flow.

- Urinate while standing on the front part of the feet, in other words, on both the balls and toes (not on the toes alone).
- Keep your teeth clenched together, but not too hard, for the entire time as you urinate.
- When you have finished urinating, lower your heels to the floor; at the same time, exhale and relax.

The secret of this method is that it increases urine flow and thereby activates kidney energy through pressure on an important energy point.

One way to determine sexual strength is to observe the force of your urine flow: a very strong flow means great sexual strength; a very weak flow, which in extreme cases may amount only to dribbles, indicates that sexual strength has declined. The simple fact that urine flow is stronger before sexual intercourse than after would tend to confirm this theory.

Massaging the three yin trajectories

Sit on the ground, with your legs spread as wide apart as possible. Begin massaging your calves and inner thighs in an upward direction only (that is, toward the groin), by rubbing the skin of your legs vigorously with your hands.

When your hands reach the groin, run them down along your leg very gently—applying almost no pressure at all—until you reach the ankle.

Do this at least thirty times on each side. Then lie down on the floor for a minute and relax.

The recumbent Taoist's exercise

This exercise was originally used to treat lumbago, but because it firms up the waist and strengthens the abdominal muscles, it can also increase sexual strength through its local stimulating action. This method also increases the energy of the kidneys, which are involved in these movements as well. The exercise consists of six separate movements. Perform each movement at least three times.

1. Lie on your back, stretched out on the floor; lift both legs straight up off the floor until they are perpendicular to the floor. Then, bring your legs down to the left, lowering them slowly until they just touch the floor. Bring them back up to the center, and perform the same movement again, this time to the right. Repeat two more times.

2. Lying on your back, raise both legs so that they are at a forty-five-degree angle to the floor. Keeping the leg muscles tensed, cross and uncross your legs three times, then gently lower them as you exhale.

3. Lying on your back, your palms flat against the floor alongside your waist, raise your upper body while inhaling (inhale naturally, without forcing the breath); then lower your upper body slowly to the floor as you exhale. Perform this movement at least three times.

4. Lying on your belly, with both hands folded alongside your head, raise your lower body and your arms at the same time.

5. Lying on your belly, with your arms behind your back, hands touching, raise your upper body and your legs at the same time.

6. Lying on your belly, raise one leg then the other. Repeat several times.

These excercises are not recommended for people with hardening of the arteries or high blood pressure.

The Red Dragon
The Red Dragon method consists of a series of traditional Taoist exercises combined with massage. It is designed to increase a man's sexual capacities and enable him to keep

an erection during long sexual intercourse. The Red Dragon method stimulates *jing* and *qi* while fortifying *shen*. Thus, each of the three treasures benefits from this practice, which, though quite simple, requires some attention at first. Mastering the Red Dragon method requires regular practice and perseverance. But after a month or so of practice, you will only have to perform this exercise once a day to maintain its benefits.

The Red Dragon, which involves movements of the penis and the muscles surrounding the anus, mobilizes muscles rarely used in daily life. These exercises are supplemented with massages designed to stimulate and tone certain parts of the body. Assiduous practice of the Red Dragon method can prevent premature ejaculation. By allowing you to control ejaculation, it will help your partner achieve orgasm as well. To obtain definite results, these exercises generally need to be performed three times a day. Don't expect immediate results. It takes time, but eventually you will see the effects.

Just before beginning each sequence, relax completely. Let your thoughts rest and observe your breathing while keeping your eyes gently shut.

- Kneel on the floor. Your toes and the tops of your feet should be in contact with the floor, the soles facing upward toward the sky. Your knees should be two to four palm widths apart to ensure proper stability.
- Take your scrotum in your left hand and squeeze gently seven times. Each squeeze should last about a second.
- Then exhale gently through your mouth until there is almost no air left in your lungs. Then inhale slowly through your nose, imagining your breath traveling

down toward your *dantian*, about three thumb widths below the navel.

- The intake of breath should last about five seconds (but in no case should be forced). Once the *dantian* is full, hold your breath. Then, with the tip of the index finger of your right hand, press the *huiyin* acupuncture point, located midway between your anus and your scrotum, and clench your teeth together gently. Place your tongue against the back of your upper front teeth, where the teeth meet the gums, thus connecting two important channels—the *Du Mai* and *Ren Mai*.

- Firmly contract the muscles of your anus, bringing it toward the front of your body, and, with your back straight, bend your upper body forward about thirty degrees while keeping your abdominal muscles contracted (but without forcing them). Then raise your buttocks about four inches above your heels.

- Hold this position for about five seconds, keeping your back straight and your anus contracted. Then let your anus relax, and then relax your entire body, the nerves and muscles. At the same time, start exhaling, letting the air escape first through your nose, then through your mouth.

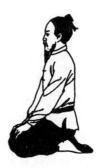

The Red Dragon: first position.

The movements of the Red Dragon method described above constitute one complete cycle. Perform the cycle twenty times. In performing these movements, you should aim for a certain fluidity, which will come eventually with practice. The Red Dragon is best practiced on awaking or just before going to bed. One sign of success is for your penis to stand up on its own when you contract your anus, as though your penis were increasing in volume.

STRENGTHENING SEXUALITY THROUGH MOXIBUSTION

Moxibustion is a separate Chinese and Taoist therapeutic method. It is easily learned because it is applied according to symptomatic principles. For all types of fatigue and energy or blood deficiency, moxibustion is the method of choice for strengthening the energies.

Here are some important things to remember if you decide to practice moxibustion on yourself, either as a remedy or for strengthening the energies:

- Start this method during a waxing moon. (Refer to a calendar to determine the lunar periods: the dark disk represents the beginning of a waxing moon and the white disk its end.)

- Perform this method only in the morning. (It is easiest to set yang in motion naturally at this time and also when the moon is waxing.)

- Use only moxa sticks (not cones) in order to avoid the risk of burns from the direct application of the moxas. These sticks represent an indirect and gentle form of moxibustion. When using these sticks, you don't actually touch the skin itself; instead, you merely warm the acupuncture point for a certain period of time and from a distance.

- Use Nian-Ying or Tai-Yi moxibustion sticks, which are made in Shanghai.

- Be sure to follow the method regularly, every day for at least ten days. Stop the treatment for three weeks, then begin again, one week a month until the desired result is obtained.

- Treat the indicated points using the following toning method: Hold the burning moxa several centimeters from the skin to produce a hot, but pleasant sensation, without any burning feeling. Hold the moxa at this distance for about five to ten minutes without moving it.

THE SEVEN MOXIBUSTION POINTS FOR STRENGTHENING MALE SEXUAL ENERGIES

Mingmen: The Vital Gate

Use moxas to tonify the *mingmen* point (GV4). This point, the Vital Gate, tones original *jing* energy and the kidneys, balances the sperm, stops vaginal emissions in women, harmonizes blood, and promotes the flow of energy in the channels of the entire body. Moxibustion at this point is also indicated for infertility.

The *mingmen* point, on the *Du* channel, is located between the kidneys on the posterior midline, in the hollow just below the spinous process of the second lumbar vertebra. Massaging this point tones the kidneys, strengthens sexual potency, and balances the vital energy of the stomach and spleen.

Zongmen

This point is located on the *Ren* channel, along the midline of the abdomen, four millimeters above the navel. Located in the center of the stomach, it is useful in treating gastric problems, toning the spleen, balancing the vital energy of the stomach, and regularizing the Middle Burner. Daily massage of this point can yield satisfactory results in cases of sexual problems of digestive origin.

Zhangmen

This point, located on the side of the abdomen, below the tip of the eleventh floating rib, is useful for activating the circulation of blood, toning the spleen, and unblocking the channels. It is particularly useful in treating sexual problems such as seminal emissions and impotence.

Qihai

The *qihai* point lies on the *Ren* channel, on the anterior midline of the lower abdomen, one and a half thumb widths below the navel. Moxibustion of the *qihai* aids in the treatment of ailments stemming from weak vital energy—seminal emissions, and, in women, vaginal discharges and irregular menstrual periods; it can also prevent physical debilitation.

Guanyan

This point, which some people call *cimen* or *dantian*, also lies on the *Ren* channel. It is located on the anterior midline of the lower abdomen, three thumb widths below the navel. It can fortify not only sexual functions but one's general physical constitution. It is particularly useful in treating ailments caused by asthenia, such as asthma, enuresis (urinary incontinence), seminal emissions, impotence, hernia, hematuria, abdominal pains, and diarrhea.

Xinshu

Xinshu, on the urinary bladder channel of *taiyang*, is located on the back, below the spinous process of the fifth dorsal vertebra, 1.5 millimeters from the posterior midline. This point is useful in treating disorders such as seminal emissions, angina pectoris, spitting up of blood, vomiting, melancholia, hemiplegia, poor memory, irritability, and fainting (due to fear). Moxibustion of this point calms the spirit, unblocks the channels, regularizes vital energy and blood, tones the muscles, and fortifies the bones.

Zusanli

This point is located on the lateral-front side of the leg, three thumb widths below the *Dubi* point, the width of an index finger from the front edge of the tibia. *Zusanli* lies on the stomach channel of foot-*yangmin*. Moxibustion of this point is useful for strengthening one's physical constitution, regularizing vital energy, toning the stomach and spleen, combating breathing impairments, and unblocking the channels. It is also effective in treating ailments such as physical debilitation, nausea, diarrhea, and dizziness, as well as sexual troubles caused by renal weaknesses. In women, it can treat atrophy of the vulva.

SEXUAL TONING THROUGH ACUPRESSURE

Acupressure is a toning massage that is useful in treating the following ailments: weakness or insufficiency of vital energy, lowered resistance to infection, weakness of the physiological functions, sexual disorders, and fragile health in older persons.

When using acupressure for sexual toning, you should apply sufficient pressure to achieve a slight feeling of stimulation; massage in the direction of the blood flow, toward the heart; and massage in a clockwise direction. Treatment with acupressure consists of mild toning, three times a week, of the acupuncture points listed below. These points can be found in any anatomical acupuncture atlas.

Male impotence: Governing Vessel 4 (GV4), Bladder 23,

GV2, Conception Vessel 3 (CV3), Stomach 36, Spleen 6, Large Intestine 5, Heart 7.

Premature ejaculation: Use these two treatments in alternation: (1) CV4, Kidney 3, Stomach 36; (2) Bladder 23, Bladder 52, Spleen 6.

Male sterility: Bladder 23 (the twenty-third point on the bladder channel tones the kidneys), GV4. It is also recommended that you sleep at night with your hands cupping your testicles.

YANG JI-ZHOU'S SYMPTOM POINTS

The following points are mentioned in a number of ancient treatises on acupuncture, including Yang Ji-zhou's sixteenth-century work, *Compendium of Acupuncture and Moxibustion.* These points can be used either to complement other energy methods or alone, as long as they do not disrupt the interplay of the energies.

Male sterility: Tone Bladder 23.

Sexual anhedonia (lack of pleasure during sex): Tone Stomach 45.

Fear of the opposite sex: Tone Kidney 5.

Retarded orgasm: Tone Stomach 15 (according to the *Yi Cheu,* a classic work on acupuncture).

Postorgasmic fatigue (in women): Tone Bladder 33 (according to the *Da Cheng*).

Incomplete erections: Tone GV1.

To increase sexual excitement for both partners during intercourse: Massage Spleen 12, located on either side of the body, in the middle of the fold of the groin.

CHAPTER TWO

The Female Sexual Tao

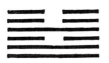

A SEXUAL problem rarely occurs in isolation. It takes form within a specific energy totality, a sort of syndrome or symptom complex. Traditional Chinese medicine recognizes a number of these sexually related syndromes, some of which are described below. Fortunately, a single individual rarely manifests all the symptoms of a given symptom complex. Nonetheless, the presence of a few of these symptoms makes it possible to identify a syndrome, determine its pathological tendencies, and thus avert them.

FEMALE SEXUAL FATIGUES

Deficiency of kidney yin
Signs: Protracted illness, insomnia, night sweats, dry mouth, dry throat, aching in the heels and lumbar region.
Sexual manifestation: Profuse and incessant anovulatory uterine bleeding.

Deficiency of kidney yang
Signs: Aversion to cold, pallor.
Sexual manifestation: Clear vaginal discharge, infertility due to cold in the uterus.

Deficiency of kidney yin and yang

Signs: Dizziness; ringing in the ears (tinnitus); aching and weakness in the lumbar region and knee joints; profuse, dilute urine.

Sexual manifestation: Vaginal discharge, infertility.

Deficiency of *jin* and kidney *qi*

Signs: Old age or *lao-sun* (fatigue with exhaustion); frequent micturation with pale, dilute urine, becoming more pronounced at night with each urination; sometimes accompanied by urinary incontinence.

Sexual manifestation: Clear, watery vaginal discharge.

Depletion of kidney jing

Signs: Weak constitution, overtiredness, chronic illness, dizziness, and ringing in the ears.

Sexual manifestation: Infertility.

Deficiency of spleen and kidney yang

Signs: Cold limbs, pallor, weight loss, mental fatigue, cold and pain in the abdomen, diarrhea with pale stools, diarrhea in the early morning, cold and aching in the lower back and knee joints, frequent micturation with dribbling and urgency, frequent nighttime urination or dysuria (difficulties in urinating).

Sexual manifestation: Infertility due to cold in the uterus, clear vaginal discharge.

Deficiency of lung and kidney yin

Signs: Unproductive cough, dry mouth, dry throat, hoarseness, aching and weakness in the lumbar region and knee joints, nervous agitation, disturbed sleep patterns, a feeling of heat emanating from the bones, intermittent fever, night sweats, flushed cheeks.

Sexual manifestation: Exacerbated and unrestrained sexual activity.

FRIGIDITY AND THE BODY'S ENERGIES

The energy imbalances discussed above can all provoke sexual difficulties, especially frigidity. When the woman's sexual functions are normal and she has an acceptable sexual partner, her vagina should lubricate sufficiently, and she should be able to have orgasm occasionally and feel pleasure during sexual intercourse.

A recurrent and persistent absence of lubrication, vaginal dilation, and orgasm is the sign of sexual troubles or frigidity. Taoists think that the problems a woman can have in producing sufficient lubrication or attaining orgasm are not psychological in origin but result from a uterus that is, in a real and concrete way, too cold. The term for female frigidity in traditional Chinese medicine is "cold womb," and the only way to put an end to it is to "warm the uterus" by attending to the underlying energies.

Treatments of female sexual deficiencies often involve a comparison between human sexuality and the interaction of fire and water. When a woman's vagina lacks lubrication prior to the sex act, it means that she is suffering from a deficiency of kidney yin; the absence of vaginal dilation is due to a deficiency of kidney yang. Under these conditions, the uterus retracts because its temperature is too low and the fluids are obstructed. These phenomena, originating in an energy imbalance, can lead to indifference toward or even fear of or disgust for sexual relations on the part of the woman.

The deficiencies of the body always have some sexual manifestation. Here are some examples:

Deficiency of the kidneys: Joint pains; weakness in the legs; profuse urine; scanty menstrual flow; lack of sexual desire; infertility; slow, deep pulse; thin, light coating on the tongue.

Deficiency of blood: Pale or dull complexion; dry skin; weakness; abnormal menstruation; infertility; weak, thready pulse; whitish tongue.

Deficiency of yang: Cold in the lower abdomen and the lumbar region; lower abdominal pains; abnormal menstruation; deep, slow pulse.

Deficiency of kidney yin and liver congestion: Inexplicable crying, irritability, hysteria, mood swings, yawning, irregular appetite, dry stools.

All of these troubles are of course accompanied by a lack of desire for sex, or frigidity.

PLANTS AND FEMALE SEXUALITY

Here are a few plants known for their stimulating effect on female sexuality:

CHINESE ANGELICA: A TRUE FEMALE TONIC

Chinese angelica (Danggui) is regarded as the female equivalent of ginseng. The root of this plant contains substances that are similar in composition to female hormones. It is widely used in China in the months following childbirth to restore the vital forces and balance the blood. Chinese angelica is not recommended for use during pregnancy, however, because it tones the uterus. It is very useful for symptoms of menopause, including hot flashes, depression, aggressiveness, headaches, and joint pains. Some Chinese herbalists recommend the use of Chinese angelica for two-week health cures twice a year, preferably in spring and autumn.

If we open the Chinese encyclopedia of medicinal plants, we will find under the rubric of Chinese angelica the following explanations:

Botanical reference: Chinese angelica.
Chinese name: Danggui.
Part used: Dried root.
Recommended dose: Four to eight grams a day.
Energy: Warm.
Taste: Sweet and pungent.
Actions: Tones the blood, activates the circulation of blood, regulates menstruation, relieves rheumatic pains.
Indications: Female sexual fatigue, frigidity, anemia, irregular or painful menstruation, vaginal bleeding, postpartum abdominal pains, constipation due to deficiency of blood, infertility.
Home use of Chinese angelica: In certain Chinese grocery stores, you can find it in a manufactured preparation under the name Dang Gui Gin, an angelica-based liquid tonic of high quality.
Administration: Regardless of format (liquid, root, syrup, pills), Chinese angelica should be taken about thirty

minutes before each of the three main meals with a little water that has been boiled and then allowed to cool until tepid. This will aid the absorption of the angelica by the intestine.

Here is a traditional Taoist method for the Chinese angelica cure. This cure, to be taken in spring or autumn, should last two weeks.

- Every day for two weeks drink two glasses of Chinese angelica decoction.
- For two glasses of the decoction, cook slowly, using a double boiler, six grams of cut-up Chinese angelica root in five to six cups of water for three hours.
- Cook in a clay or earthenware pot.

This cure will fortify your ovaries and Fallopian tubes. Chinese angelica can help your body to maintain its production of estrogen well into old age and thus can delay the onset of menopause and retard the aging process. Many therapists recommend this cure as a preventive measure for women in good health. The prevention of disease has always been a top priority for natural medicine.

ALOE: GREEN GOLD

Botanical reference: Aloe vera.
Energy: Cool.
Taste: Bitter.
Actions: Relieves constipation, unblocks the liver and the bile ducts, regulates menstruation, rejuvenates the body, fortifies and beautifies the female sexual organs.
Properties: Laxative, vulnerary, emollient, emmenagogic.

Energy profile: Apparently of Persian origin, aloe is highly esteemed by Chinese therapists. Medical treatises from China and India consider it the herb of choice for treating constipation and scanty, irregular, and painful menstruation.

Utilization: Used alone, aloe can trigger diarrhea, which is why Indian therapists mix it with a little ginger. This mixture has the further advantage of reducing the nausea that some people experience when swallowing aloe. The aloe plant is well adapted to temperate climates and can be grown in a backyard garden without too much trouble. It is used as part of the regenerative cures (*Rasayana*) of the yogi doctors of south India, who believe that constipation is the mother of all illnesses and aging; their rejuvenating cures are designed to rid the body of toxins and prevent their further accumulation. "The aloe cure," certain Taoists claim, "preserves youth and vigor and thus promotes longevity." Taoist physicians also use aloe to fortify the brain, decongest the liver, and encourage the growth of hair. According to scientists, the abundant presence of vitamin A in aloe accounts for some of its revitalizing properties, which have been widely recognized since antiquity.

Administration: According to the Taoist tradition, the usual daily dose consists of four grams of powdered aloe leaves (available from herbalist pharmacies) mixed together with two grams of powdered ginger root and a teaspoon of good-quality honey. Take half of this mixture on awaking and the rest at night, before bedtime. Continue this cure for one week while eliminating mutton, fish, and sesame oil from your diet. Ideally, one should eat a vegetarian diet for the entire week, with lots of white rice (brown rice would be too irritating to the intestines). If you find the taste of aloe disagreeable, you can take two gel capsules three times a day before meals.

RASPBERRY LEAVES

Botanical reference: Rubus idaeus.
Energy: Cold.
Taste: Astringent.
Actions: Harmonizes pregnancy; relieves menstrual pain, stomach troubles, and symptoms of menopause.
Properties: Diuretic, depurative, astringent, emmenagogic, antiscorbutic.
Energy profile: Chinese physicians, who have long recognized these properties in the raspberry, consider it a veritable panacea for female disorders, such as painful menstruation, vaginal discharges, and symptoms of menopause. Curiously enough, obstetricians during World War II discovered that fragarine, the active agent in raspberry leaves, is a relaxant for the muscles of the uterus.
Administration: The best way to use raspberry leaves (available from herbalist pharmacies) is in a concentrated infusion, which can be prepared in the following manner: Take fifty grams of the plant and cover with a liter of boiling water. Cover the vessel (preferably a clay pot) and let infuse ten minutes. Strain. Drink three cups of this infusion every day for several weeks. Raspberry-leaf extract can also be used, two tablespoons diluted in a little warm water, three times a day. However, the alcohol in the extract can have a negative effect on sensitive livers, and this treatment should not be used for an extended period of time. A decoc-

tion of raspberry leaves with a little witch hazel makes a good vaginal douche, useful in treating leukorrhea. This cure should be halted as soon as the discharges cease.

CLASSIC TAOIST FORMULAS FOR STRENGTHENING FEMALE SEXUALITY

Listed below are the traditional medicinal formulas that are most appropriate for treating female sexual problems. Their composition is precise, and they can be prepared by specialized herbalists as either decoctions or soluble powders. Follow the herbalist's instructions as to the proper dose.

Fertility-promoting pill
Zan Yu Dan
Composition: Aconite carmichaeli, Herba Cistanchis desedicolae, Epimedium grandiflora (Yin Yang Huo), *Allium sativum* (Da Suan), *Cornus officinalis* (Shan Zhu Yu), *Rehmannia praeparata* (Shou Di Huang), *Lycium sinensis* (Gou Qi Zi), *Cinnamomum cassia* (Rou Gui), *Morinda officinalis* (Ba Ji Tian), fructus *Cnidii Monnieri*, Rh *Curculiginis orchioidis, Eucommia ulminoides* (Du Zhong), *Angelica sinensis* (Dang Gui), *Atractylodes macrocephala* (Bai Zhu).
Actions: Tones and warms the kidneys.
General indications: Depletion of kidney yang (insufficiency of *mingmen* fire) and depletion of *yuanqi*, apathy, lack of determination, lumbago, weakness in the lumbar area, pallor.
Sexual indications: Infertility, frigidity due to a "cold uterus."
Format and administration: For boluses, reduce the ingredients to a powder, then add a little honey and form pills

the size of green peas. Three to six grams a day in two to three doses with a little hot water. In decoction, sixty to one hundred grams per liter. Reduce to forty centiliters. Take this amount over the course of a day in three to four doses.

Lower-back-fortifying and kidney-strengthening tablet

Yao Jian Shen Pian

Composition: Rhizoma *Cibotii barometz, Eucommia ulminoides* (Du Zhong), *Loranthus parasiticus* (Sang Ji Sheng), *Poria cocos* (Fu Ling), caulis *Millettiae reticulatae,* fructus *Rosae, Laevigatate sclerotium, Cordyceps sinensis,* fructus *Rubi chingii.*

Actions: Tones kidney *qi* and yang, strengthens the sinews and bones.

General indications: Depletion of kidney yang; chronic nephritis; lumbago; weakness in the lumbar region, waist, and knee joints; lower-back pain; vertigo; tinnitus; frequent, scanty urination, with dribbling; dyspnea; poor memory; fatigue.

Sexual indications: Fatigue following sexual excesses.

Format and administration: Pills, in bottles of one hundred (United Pharmaceutical Manufactory, Guangzhou, Guangdong). Four pills, once or twice a day, with a little warm water.

COMMERCIALLY MANUFACTURED FORMULAS FOR FEMALE SEXUALITY

Pills of commercial manufacture can be either classic formulas or a single herb prepared for mass-market consumption. The following are formulas with sexual actions:

Royal Jelly
Feng Wang Jiang

Actions: Tones the Triple Burner and the kidneys, tones yin and *qi*, promotes fertility and longevity (particularly recommended for women). Maintains the sexual fluids and the beauty of the sexual organs.

General indications: Weight loss, senility, general debilitation, convalescence, hair loss, neurasthenia, hepatitis, arthritis, anemia, postsurgical treatment in cases of gastric ulcers.

Recommended dosage: One to two vials per day.

Chinese Angelica Pill
Dang Gui Wan

Actions: Activates and nourishes the circulation of blood, soothes pains, lubricates the intestines, relieves tensions.

Indications: Deficiency of blood after childbirth; menstrual disorders such as dysmenorrhea, amenorrhea, scanty menstruation, headaches; lumbago; abdominal swelling; gynecopathy; traumatisms; constipation; dry skin; eruptions.

Sexual indications: Weak feminine energy.

Recommended dosage: Two to five pills, three times a day.

Heart-Supplementing and Spirit-Quieting Pill
Tian Wang Pu Xin Tan

Actions: Nourishes tired heart, calms emotional instability.

General indications: Lassitude, anxiety, ringing in the ears, palpitations, breathing difficulties, insomnia, poor memory, night sweats.

Sexual indications: Mental fatigue, sexual difficulties due to anxiety.

Recommended dosage: Five pills, three times a day.

NOURISHING SEXUALITY THROUGH DIET

Taoist culture recognizes the utility of certain foods for the maintenance of good health. Some of these belong to the category of tonics. These foods, as one might expect, stimulate the sexual functions.

Here are some foods that are recognized for their sexual properties. They are particularly useful in cases of sexual fatigue and frigidity:

FOOD	ENERGY ACTION
Red dates	Tones energy (qi)
Raspberry leaves	Tones the blood
Wheat germ	Tones the heart
Black soybeans	Activates the blood and promotes the flow of fluids
Longan	Tones the blood
Honey	Relieves dryness through lubricating action (develops secretions)
Licorice	Tones energy (qi)
Black sesame	Relieves dryness through humidifying action (develops secretions)
Red wine	Tones the blood (when used in small quantities)

SIMPLIFIED DIETARY RECOMMENDATIONS FOR SEXUAL DEFICIENCIES

The Taoist dietary recommendations in the previous chapter on male sexuality are effective in treating female sexual problems as well. Foods for treating impotence in men can be used to treat frigidity in women. The following information completes the picture for women.

Deficiency of the kidneys

Indications: Joint pains; weakness in the legs; profuse urine; scanty menstrual flow; lack of sexual desire; infertility; slow, deep pulse; thin, light coating on the tongue.

Traditional Taoist dietary recommendation: Warm the energy of the kidneys and that of the Conception Vessel with fennel decoction, dill, mutton.

Deficiency of blood

Indications: Pale or dull complexion; dry skin; weakness; abnormal menstruation; infertility; weak, thready pulse; whitish tongue.

Traditional Taoist dietary recommendation: Nourish the blood and humidify the kidneys with egg yolks, cuttlefish, nutmeg (in small quantities), raw oysters, spinach.

Deficiency and cold in the sexual organs (cold uterus)

Indications: Cold in the lower abdomen and lower back; lower abdominal pains; menstrual trouble; deep, slow pulse.

Traditional Taoist dietary recommendation: Soy milk, capers, cooked endives, frog legs, old red wine (Bordeaux), lamb, fresh goat's milk.

Deficiency of kidney yin and liver congestion

Indications: Inexplicable crying, irritability, hysteria, mood swings, yawning, irregular appetite, dry stools.

Traditional Taoist dietary recommendation: Decongest the liver channel and humidify the kidneys with the following foods: pear peelings, asparagus, coconut milk, duck, mulberries, raw oysters, decoction of orange peels, and flowers and leaves of the mandarin orange tree.

All of these troubles are of course accompanied by a lack of sexual appetite, or frigidity.

SIMPLE RECIPES FOR FEMALE SEXUALITY AND FEMININE BEAUTY

Here are a few Taoist recipes intended to supplement and improve the sexual energies. They are based on alimentary energy principles and on the interplay of the five flavors.

Wheat soup
Indications: Menopause, hot flashes, night sweats.
Counter-indications: Aversion to cold.
Ingredients: 60 grams wheat (Fu Xiao Mai), 30 grams lily bulb, 10 grams licorice, 10 grams jujube.
Preparation: Soak all ingredients in 450 milliliters of water for 1 hour. Boil for 35 minutes over a low flame. Strain, reserving only the liquid.
Drink this juice in two doses every day during the daytime for fifteen days.

Rice with polygonatum
Indications: Menopause, dizziness, hot flashes.
Counter-indications: Aversion to cold.
Ingredients: 30 grams polygonatum root (Huang Jin), 30 grams polygoni root (Shou Wu), 50 grams white rice.
Actions: The tuber of *Polygonatum multiflorum* is a major blood tonic and a major kidney yin tonic. In Chinese herbal medicine, it is considered to have a sweet flavor, warm energy, and an astringent nature, which makes it a good remedy for diarrhea. This plant is especially useful for treating yin deficiencies of the kidneys and the liver, char-

acterized by blackouts or dizzy spells, premature graying of the hair, lumbago, and vaginal discharges. Polygonatum tones blood and the kidneys.

Preparation: Soak the polygonatum and polygoni roots in 500 milliliters of water for an hour. Boil for 30 minutes. Strain, reserving only the liquid. Cook the rice in the strained liquid for 20 minutes over a low flame.

Eat twice weekly for a month.

Wormwood soup

This dish contains eggs, which tone the blood and increase the level of iron in the blood.

Indications: Painful menstruation, excessive menstrual flow, anemia due to excessive menstrual flow.

Counter-indications: Sweating, fever, thirst.

Preparation: Put the wormwood leaves into a pot with 250 milliliters of water. Boil for 20 minutes. Strain, reserving the liquid and discarding the leaves. Into the liquid, break two eggs, add some sugar, and boil.

Wormwood leaves warm and tone the energy channels, including the Governing Vessel and the Conception Vessel. Eat this soup in two portions, both during the daytime, for two days during your menstrual period.

Ginseng and Chinese angelica soup

Indications: Menstrual pains, insufficiency of energy and of blood, shortness of breath, palpitations.

Counter-indications: Periods with heavy clotting.

Ingredients: 20 grams Chinese angelica root, 10 grams ginseng root, 30 grams astragalus root, 15 grams jujube fruit, 60 grams lotus seeds, 50 grams white rice.

Preparation: Split the lotus seed in two and remove the kernel. Hull the jujubes and cut the astragalus root into slices.

Soak all the ingredients, except the rice, in a liter of water for 2 hours. Boil for 10 minutes, then remove the astragalus slices. Add the rice and cook over a low flame for 20 minutes.

Eat twice a week for a month.

Mandarin orange leaf tea

Indications: Premenstrual swelling of the breasts and bloating, irregular periods, clotting, obstruction of liver energy, intense menstrual pains.

Actions: The leaves of the mandarin orange tree unblock liver energy and have a calming effect. The twigs of the perilla tree improve the circulation of energy.

Preparation: Place all ingredients in a pot. Pour 250 milliliters of boiling water over them and cover for 15 minutes. Strain.

Use: Drink as a tea during the day. Follow this treatment for five days before the onset of your period and for five days after.

Decoction of licorice, wheat, and dates

Ingredients: 10 grams licorice, 1 teaspoon wheat germ, 5 pitted red dates.

Actions: Treats female psychological problems such as hysteria and anxiety, which can cause frigidity.

Preparation: Place all the ingredients in a pot. Pour 250 milliliters of boiling water over them and boil gently for 15 minutes. Strain.

Use: Drink as a tea during the daytime for ten days before your period.

Black soybeans, black sesame, and honey

Ingredients: 1 tablespoon black soybeans, 1 tablespoon black sesame seeds, 1 tablespoon honey.

Actions: Stimulates the circulation of blood in the lower abdomen, increases vaginal secretions.

Preparation: Place the soybeans and the sesame seeds in a pot, and pour 250 milliliters of boiling water over them. Boil for 15 minutes over a low flame. Strain. Let the mixture cool to lukewarm, then add 1 tablespoon of honey.

Use: Drink as a tea, during the daytime for three weeks.

Raspberry wine

Ingredients: Raspberry leaves, red wine.

Actions: Tones and purifies the blood, develops vaginal secretions.

Preparation: Add a handful of raspberry leaves to 1 liter of good red wine. Close the bottle and let steep for at least three weeks in a cool, dark place.

Longan wine

Ingredients: Longans, red wine, honey.

Actions: Longan has a sweet taste and hot energy. It is a major blood tonic and is used as an energy tonic, particularly by pregnant women and older persons. This preparation tones the sexual fluids and strengthens the female sexual organs. Legend has it that in ancient China, a woman with a taste for this wine drank it in large quantities; its fabulous properties made her the most beautiful woman in all Chinese history. In many regions of China, local healers and herbalists consider longans a beauty secret and sexual tonic.

Preparation: Longan wine can be prepared in the following manner: Place 150 grams of longans in a large vessel and add 4 tablespoons of red wine. Boil over a low flame for 20 minutes. Remove from heat and let cool. Transfer to a bottle containing 2 liters of wine. Add a little honey and seal the bottle, letting it rest for a month in a dark place.

Longan decoction to tone the blood

Ingredients: Longans, water.

Actions: This formula is particularly useful for women suffering from deficiency of blood and deficiency of heart energy, with symptoms such as palpitations, especially during the night, accompanied by sweating, nervousness, and anxiety. Bestows a healthy coloring and beautiful skin. Also relieves palpitations, night sweats, nervousness, and anxiety.

Preparation: 25 grams of longans, the roots removed, in a container with half a bowl of water. Boil over a low flame for 20 minutes.

EXERCISES FOR STRENGTHENING FEMALE SEXUALITY

Most female sexual troubles—irregular or painful periods, leukorrhea, frigidity—can be attributed to an imbalance of vital energy and blood. These internal exercises tone the energy of the lower abdomen while respecting the female yin essence.

The three exercises of the wild duck

Many of the energy channels are involved in sexually related disorders. These channels include the kidney, liver, and spleen channels and the Conception Vessel. For this reason it is necessary to establish a general exercise program

THE TAO OF LOVE

to fortify all these channels and to regularize the circulation of blood to prevent blood stases and weakness of the blood (anemia). This short sequence of exercises can be practiced any time of the day. It is easily memorized. The movements come directly from the *qigong*, the Chinese system of health exercises.

These movements are of ancient origin. Long ago, many years before the birth of Christ, the renowned physician Hua To used acupuncture theory to devise a series of movements that imitated the movements of animals. His purpose was to stimulate the weak energy from which members of the Chinese imperial court were suffering.

If it was recognized even then that a sedentary lifestyle could be harmful for health, what about today? These ancient and traditional exercises have recently been taken up again in China and Japan. They are specially designed to tighten the skin, combat obesity and cellulite, slim the waist, and, above all, fortify the female sexual organs. By practicing these exercises regularly, you can lose weight, become slimmer, more relaxed, and more svelte, and improve the functioning of your sexual organs.

These exercises are best practiced in the sequence indicated. In performing these exercises, be sure not to force any of the movements. Perform them slowly and deliberately, and don't let yourself get distracted. Repeat each movement no more than five times.

First exercise: Stand on the balls and toes of your feet and raise your arms while stretching upward and inhaling gently. Then lower your body and bring your arms down; while still keeping your heels off the floor, exhale gently until there is no more air in your lungs. Lower your head, bringing it down between your knees. Then stand up again on the balls and toes of your feet and repeat the entire movement four more times.

This exercise invigorates the torso, the sides especially, at the level of the rib cage. It also increases lung capacity and brings oxygen to every part of the body, helping to maintain the proper functioning of the organs and improving elimination. It stimulates circulation in the pelvic region and the sexual organs.

Second exercise: Sit on the floor with your legs extended in front of you, your weight principally on your buttocks. Let your hands rest on your legs. Exhale gently as you slowly bring your head down to your legs and try to touch your feet with your hands. Inhale as you return to the original position, keeping your arms extended. (If you feel too much pulling in your back or in the back of your legs during this exercise, you can let your hands stay near your knees rather than try to touch your toes. The important thing is to keep your legs extended.)

This movement will restore beauty and svelteness to your midriff and abdomen. It refines the tissues and tones the internal organs.

Third exercise: Sitting on the floor, balance yourself on your buttocks while supporting yourself with your extended arms. With your legs extended, describe five circles in space in a clockwise direction; then, in a counterclockwise direction, make five more circles. Keeping your feet together will make it easier to rotate your extended legs.

In the beginning, two circles may be all you can do before you tire. If that happens, gradually increase the number of circles over the course of time until you can do five of them. Make these circles gently while breathing in a natural, unforced manner.

This movement refines and tones the muscles of the buttocks and the hips. It promotes the elimination of fat from the back and the hips. It is also excellent for sagging buttocks.

Daoyin for female sexuality

The *daoyin* method for directing energy, described in the previous chapter on the male sexual Tao, can be profitably practiced by women, too; it treats kidney deficiencies and increases vital energy in the pubic and genital region. Perform this exercise in exactly the same way as indicated in the previous chapter.

Method for controlling the vagina

Just as there are specific exercises for the male sexual organs, so there are methods for controlling the energies of the vagina. The ancient Taoists developed a method designed to strengthen and maintain the vaginal muscles with a sequence of alternating contractions and relaxations. This method can be practiced anywhere and anytime; it should always be performed in a standing position, with the tip of your tongue placed behind your upper front teeth, where the teeth meet the gums. This will allow you to connect two of the "extra channels," the *Du Mai* and the *Ren Mai*, so as to form a complete yin-yang energy circuit, sometimes called the wheel of fortune.

This method is commonly used in certain types of Chinese Taoist and Indian tantric meditation. The vaginal control exercise is performed in the following way:

Breathe in through your nose, and with each inhalation, raise your tongue to the roots of your teeth while contracting your vaginal-anal region and bringing it upward. Exhale through your mouth, and with each exhalation relax your anus and vagina, while also letting your tongue relax and rest on the floor of your mouth.

This exercise offers many benefits: it activates energy and blood, prevents genital disorders, improves a woman's ability to carry a child to term, prevents hemorrhoids, increases vaginal secretions, and enhances the response to sexual stimuli.

Breathe deeply and naturally from the abdomen while performing this exercise. Your abdomen should swell out with each inhalation and relax with each exhalation. It is a good idea to combine vaginal exercises with a gentle massaging of the ears (remember the relationship between the ears and the kidneys) and the eyes. It is said that women who are adept at performing this exercise can absorb the man's yang energy during sexual intercourse, thus helping to increase the couple's harmony.

Of all the parts of a woman's body, the vagina is probably the one most in need of exercise, followed by the anus, the ears, and the eyes. If a woman does not make a deliberate effort to exercise her vagina on a regular basis, there is little chance that it will be activated, except during her periods and during sexual relations. Consider the following: a woman uses her legs and exercises her mouth and tongue every day, as a matter of course; but she does not have her period every day or have sex every day of her life. That is why it is important for her to give her vagina special attention.

Regularly exercising the vagina and the anus has other benefits as well: it activates energy and blood circulation in

THE TAO OF LOVE

these two zones, which can shrink hemorrhoids and increase vaginal secretions.

Massage the folds of the groin

Lie flat on your back on a moderately hard surface (for example, on a carpet or rug). Relax for a few moments while focusing on your breathing, which should be slow and natural.

Then rub your hands against each other for fifteen seconds; then stop rubbing but keep the hands immobile one against the other. Repeat this action two more times, until your hands are very warm and you feel the prickly sensation that signals the presence of *qi* (vital energy).

Then start rubbing the folds of both sides of the groin, slowly and gently and without stopping. To keep your mind focused, count silently up to a hundred, then stop.

Practiced every day, in the morning upon rising and at night before going to bed, this health exercise will tone and regularize what therapists call the Elixir Field, that is, the genital hormonal system. This massage is particularly indicated for disorders of the female genital system.

MOXIBUSTION FOR THE FEMALE ENERGIES

Moxibustion is a separate Chinese and Taoist therapeutic method. It is easily learned because it is applied according to symptomatic principles. For all types of fatigue and energy or blood deficiency, moxibustion is the method of choice for strengthening the energies. For more complete information regarding the practice of moxibustion at home, refer to the previous chapter on the male sexual Tao.

THE SIX MOXIBUSTION POINTS FOR STRENGTHENING FEMALE SEXUAL ENERGY

Huiyin

Also called *pingyi*, the *huiyin* point, located on the *Ren* channel, is at the center of the perineum, between the scrotum and the anus in males and between the posterior vulva junction and the anus in females. Massaging this point, which lies at the intersection of the *Ren, Du,* and *Chong* channels, helps regularize menstruation, improves the functioning of the genital apparatus, and tones the kidneys. Moxibustion of the *huiyin* point is useful in treating such afflictions as infertility and menstrual problems and can prevent seminal emissions and premature ejaculation in men and fortify the constitution.

Shenque

Shenque, a point on the *Ren* channel, located in the middle of the abdomen, at the center of the navel, can tone the spleen, kidneys, and yang and improve the gastric and intestinal functions. *Shenque* means "traversed by the divine breath"; it is used in the treatment of infertility caused by uterine coldness and renal asthenia.

Tianshu

Also called *changxi* or *gumen*, this point is situated on the abdomen, two thumb widths to the side of the navel. It lies on the stomach channel of foot yang-*min*. Moxibustion of this point can regularize the gastric and intestinal functions and vital energy and treat female sexual problems and irregular periods.

Guanyuan

Sometimes called *cimen* or *dantian*, this point, also on the *Ren* channel, is located on the anterior midline of the lower abdomen, three thumb widths below the navel. It can fortify not only the sexual functions but the general physical constitution as well. It is particularly useful in treating ailments caused by asthenia, such as asthma, enuresis (urinary incontinence), hernia, hematuria, abdominal pains, diarrhea, irregular periods, dysmenorrhea, and hemorrhagic diathesis.

Zhongji

This point lies on the anterior midline of the lower abdomen, four millimeters below the navel. It is useful in the treatment and prevention of sexual problems. It is also useful in treating the following ailments: enuresis, hernia, urethral atresia, irregular periods, vaginal discharges, pruritis vulva (vulva itching), and asthenia of yang, and, in men, seminal emissions and impotence.

Shenshu

The *shenshu* point, on the urinary bladder channel of foot yang-*min*, is found on the lower back, below the protrusion of the second lumbar vertebra, one and a half thumb widths from the posterior midline. It is used to tone the kidneys. It is also useful in treating ailments such as enuresis, irregular periods, vaginal discharges, weakness in the lumbar region and knees, and internal lesions and general debilitation caused by overwork; in men, it helps to treat seminal emissions and impotence. Moxibustion of this point helps tone the kidneys, strengthen the constitution, improve renal function, and slow premature aging.

SEXUAL TONING THROUGH ACUPRESSURE

Acupressure is a toning massage that can treat the following ailments: weakness or insufficiency of vital energy, lowered resistance to infection, weakness of the physiological functions, sexual disorders, and fragile health in older persons.

When using acupressure for sexual tonification, you should apply sufficient pressure to achieve a slight feeling of stimulation; massage in the direction of the blood flow, toward the heart; and massage in a clockwise direction. Treatment with acupressure consists of mild toning, three times a week, of the points listed after each symptom in the following list. (For their locations, refer to any anatomical acupuncture atlas.)

Retarded orgasm: Tone Stomach 15 (according to the *Yi Cheu*, a classic work on acupuncture).

Postorgasmic fatigue: Tone Bladder 33 (according to the *Da Cheng*).

Frigidity: Tone Conception Vessel 5.

Choose three or four of the following points to tone at each session: Spleen 2, Spleen 3, Spleen 9, Bladder 23, Governing Vessel 3, Conception Vessel 6, Stomach 36, Triple Burner 5, Heart 3.

Absence of orgasm: Gently tone once a week Lung 7, Spleen 4, Liver 3, Stomach 20, Heart 6.

THE APHRODISIAC ACUPRESSURE POINT

The following point is a powerful female aphrodisiac. Located at the intersection of the Conception Vessel (*Ren Mai*) and the Governing Vessel (*Du Mai*), that is, right in the center of the perineum, between the anus and the posterior vulva junction, it is closely allied to the female sexual apparatus. In fact, ancient texts describe this point as a clitoral reflex zone. The stimulation of this point helps increase sensitivity to sexual stimuli and diminish frigidity.

Massaging this point is very simple: all you have to do is press your thumb (be sure to keep your thumbnail clipped short so that you don't injure the skin) on this point in a slightly upward direction. Apply the pressure slowly, until you just begin to feel some pain. Then release the pressure but without removing your finger from the point. Continue this cycle of pressure and release for about two minutes. Then rest and stretch out a little.

SULFUR SITZ BATH

Frequent sexual relations and conception tend to enlarge the vagina. A classic Chinese sexology text suggests a sitz bath every day for twenty days with a pinch of sulfur dissolved in warm water. "After twenty days your vagina will be the size of a virgin's."

CHAPTER THREE

The Nine Exercises of the Sexual Tao

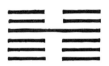

"I wanted to make love," the Yellow Emperor said, "but my penis would not become erect.

"I was ashamed to find myself like this, in a sweat before this young woman. How can I get my vigor back? Su Nu, can you give me the secrets of the sexual Tao?"

And Su Nu answered, "Your majesty, many men have this problem. When a man desires to make love, he must ready his mind and understand that the sex act needs slow, step-by-step preparation. Calmness of mind is an especially important preliminary. The man must also observe the five virtues: kindness, austerity, judicious attachment, knowledge, and sincerity."

MEN AND women of all ages can benefit from the nine exercises of the sexual Tao. These traditional exercises, which have been handed down from one generation of Taoists to the next, constitute a sort of energy calisthenics designed to preserve and optimize the sexual functions.

They not only stimulate the sexual functions but have general health benefits as well. They should be practiced every day if possible, but not within fifteen minutes before a meal or within an hour after a meal. The best times to practice these exercises are in the early morning at sunrise and—if you have the time—once again at bedtime. You can maintain the benefits of these exercises with only fifteen minutes of daily practice, but if you don't have that much time to spare, five minutes will do and is certainly better than nothing.

1. NATURAL ABDOMINAL BREATHING: THE CRANE

This breathing method is particularly beneficial for anyone who wants to begin *qigong* and for strengthening both the sexual organs and the internal organs—the stomach, intestines, liver, gall bladder, kidneys, and urinary bladder.

Staying healthy and in control of one's mental faculties means learning how to breathe deeply by developing the flexibility and tone of the abdominal muscles, particularly the diaphragm. To this end, the first Taoist physicians of ancient China invented an exercise to develop abdominal breathing. The idea for this method came to them from observing the crane, that magnificent bird, which, with its peculiar gait, always seems to be in the process of stimulating its abdomen as it walks. The exercise came to be called Crane Breathing.

Its benefits are manifold. Crane Breathing will allow you to use the movements of your diaphragm to massage your internal organs and thus improve the circulation of blood in your abdomen and genital areas. It is particularly recommended for those who suffer from chronic constipation, diarrhea, or digestive insufficiency, for the tissues of the digestive system are moved by involuntary muscles that are difficult to stimulate since they cannot easily be exercised

directly. This breathing method can also help you to increase your lung capacity appreciably; asthma sufferers and
people with chronic bronchitis can greatly benefit from it.
Crane Breathing reduces adipose tissue in the belly and
lowers cholesterol. People with hypertension will find this
exercise useful as well, because it can help decongest the
the body's upper zones.

Crane Breathing provides a good foundation for more
elaborate breathing movements. It's also a good relaxation
technique; practicing this method will give you a few precious moments every day to focus on yourself. Most people
never learn to breathe in a way that allows them to take
advantage of their full lung capacity. They never use the
lower parts of the bronchial tubes and in fact hardly ever
involve any parts of their lungs except the upper lobes.
Thus they never manage to eliminate or expel all the car-
bon dioxide and toxins that can accumulate in the blood;
as a result, their blood becomes impure and they fall ill.
That kind of insufficient breathing may be unconscious,
but it can hardly be called "natural," unlike the breathing
that we discuss here, which is also called abdominal
breathing.

Here are a number of points to keep in mind when practicing abdominal breathing: When inhaling and exhaling,
you should involve your lower abdomen. Inhalation brings
air into the bronchial tubes and fills the lungs, even the
lower parts. Once your lungs become full, they press
against the diaphragm, which consequently descends. At
that moment, the chest inflates and the abdomen swells
outward. As you exhale, your abdomen should tighten and
your diaphragm should push upward against the lungs.
This will allow the impure air to leave the lower part of

your lungs, and the movements of the lower abdomen and the diaphragm will help your lungs expand downward as well.

You can make abdominal breathing part of your normal, daily routine. Try to practice it while walking, working, or lying down. It can also become part of your meditation exercises and will facilitate normal blood circulation.

When practicing abdominal breathing, remember that your inhalations and exhalations should not be forced and the transitions from inhalation to exhalation and from exhalation to inhalation should be natural and relaxed. Unforced inhalation means inhaling gently, lightly, and effortlessly, without lifting your chest or trying to over-expand the lungs. Unforced exhalation means maintaining a gentle, effortless respiratory rhythm, without compressing your chest or flattening your stomach. The transition between inhaling and exhaling and vice versa should be light and natural, without jerkiness, tension, or interruptions.

Another aspect of Crane Breathing is known as spontaneous breathing. There are two stages of respiratory control to this "energy calisthenics." The first stage is devoted entirely to relaxation. In this stage, you pay no attention to controlling your breath. The second stage begins after you have become relaxed. At this point, you begin to regularize your breathing so that it acquires a light, smooth, and regular rhythm. As your body relaxes more and more, your respiratory movements will become gentler, lighter, and more regular in pace. And conversely, the more your breath control increases, the more you relax. During this phase, your respiratory rhythm will slacken from its normal rate of twelve to sixteen breaths per minute. A regular rhythm is well-defined and fairly constant. It should not be slow and then fast, weak and then strong, short and then long. It should be regulated consciously. By the end of this exercise, your mind will be calm and your breathing will be gentle, light, and regular.

The principal effect of abdominal breathing is to create a state of calm and tranquility. Your respiratory movements create variations of intra-abdominal pressure that massage the internal organs, and it is this massage that produces the calming effect. This internal massage has the further benefit of strengthening these organs and improving the circulation of energy and blood within and among them. The more complete your state of relaxation and the deeper your inner tranquility, the more beneficial deep breathing will be for you. That is why the first, calming stage of this exercise is so necessary.

Deep breathing is a useful treatment for people who suffer from dyspepsia or from ptoses of such organs as the stomach or kidneys. If, however, you begin to feel a sense of fullness or bloating in your abdomen, stop the exercise and return to the meditation and relaxation stage instead.

PRACTICING CRANE BREATHING

Begin by lying on the floor or on your bed. If you are on your bed, be sure to remove your pillow. Spread your legs just slightly apart, and start rubbing your hands one against the other to warm them a little. Then place your hands on your abdomen, directly on the skin, on either side of your navel.

Exhale gently and effortlessly, while pressing down with

both hands so that you make a depression in the abdomen. Expel all the air from your lungs.

Now inhale calmly, letting your belly inflate and stretch upward like a balloon filling with air. It should seem as though the air were entering your abdomen without inflating the rib cage. You can achieve this effect by gently raising your two hands, which should continue to lie flat against the area around the navel. With each inhalation, you should be conscious of this area; it is allied to the Lower Burner and the root of breath. It also represents the center of gravity around which the standing and sitting exercises that follow are structured.

Repeat this sequence of alternating inhalations and exhalations twelve times. Concentrate totally on what you are doing. You can help maintain your awareness by practicing the following visualization: imagine and feel that with each inhalation the air that is entering your body, charged with vitalizing substance and luminous *qi*, is moving downward to the lower abdomen, filling it with beneficial heat. During these internal energy exercises, feel the zones of strength as they begin to appear within the energy body.

That's all there is to it! The method is quite simple, but acquiring true mastery can take some time. After one or two weeks of practice, however, you should be feeling comfortable with this breathing technique.

This technique is the basis for a number of Chinese exercises such as Tai Chi Chuan and kung fu. Practice it in the morning when you wake up and in the evening before going to sleep. There is one exception, however: it should not be practiced by pregnant women.

Important note: When you practice Crane Breathing, you should be in a state of perfect relaxation and never force any of the movements. After mastering the relaxation techniques and spontaneous breathing, you can gradually transform spontaneous breathing into abdominal breathing. Again, the characteristics of abdominal energy breathing are as follows: your breathing rhythm should be gentle, light, regular, slow, long, and deep; on exhaling, your abdomen flattens; on inhaling, your abdomen expands.

2. UNFOLDING THE ABDOMINAL *DANTIAN*

Taoists attach great importance to the progressive development of *qi*, or vital energy. Those who would follow the Tao must first develop and purify their vital essence (*qi*) through a process called "interior alchemy." This method, which is not reserved for adepts and hermits (at least not at the level at which it is presented here), consists of developing your energy in stages. The first stage is the lighting of the abdomen's alchemical furnace, the Elixir Field, or *dantian*. As we have already pointed out, this abdominal center is closely related to sexuality, and any deficiency in this region will have sexual repercussions. Regulating the sexual functions begins with work on this center.

While the *dantian* is a definite area, it does not have a concrete anatomical location. It is an energy reservoir, and by developing it you will increase your vital force. Practically speaking, the conscious development of your *dantian* will bring healthy vitality, better digestion, a natural sexuality, and a gentle feeling of internal warmth. When the furnace has been lit, self-healing can begin.

In China there are many exercises for developing the *dan-*

tian, but it is the simplest ones that are the most effective. In this book, we have made it a point to suggest only simple and authentic methods that are accessible to everyone.

OPENING THE ABDOMINAL *DANTIAN*

Sit in a comfortable position (on the floor in a cross-legged, semi-cross-legged, or lotus position, or else on a chair). Leave your daily cares behind you and focus your awareness on feeling your body's energies.

Place one hand over the other on the abdominal cavity, just below the navel, with both palms facing the belly. Do not press too hard against the skin.

Imagine a magnificent flower, such as the golden lotus, opening its petals right in the middle of your belly. As the flower opens and its petals unfold, its warmth and perfume waft out and gradually fill your whole body, nourishing the internal organs with a blissful energy. Remain in this state for several minutes. Try to relax without falling into a state of torpor. You will begin to have sensations of heat, fullness, and distension, particularly in the belly.

Imagine the flower closing as you exhale and opening as you inhale. Your body will then begin to sway slightly, taking on a wavelike motion. Let this movement happen freely, but don't become intoxicated with it or lose control. Remain a few moments in simple contemplation of this rediscovered quietude before you once again embark on the flood of your daily activities.

Practiced once daily anytime of the day, this exercise is an excellent foundation for all Taoist meditative practices.

It's a good idea to start practicing the opening of the *dantian* for a month before you proceed to the next exercises. That way you will lay a good foundation for your daily exercise routine.

Taoists refer to this internal work as "the cultivation of *qi*." Practicing this method helps develop a sensitivity to the energy that is constantly circulating through the body. The *dantian*, that Elixir Field in the middle of our bellies just below the navel, is where the subtle energy that Taoists call ancestral energy resides. This force constitutes the human being's physical, sexual, and mental foundation. According to Taoists, it also determines how long we live. By practicing these energy-cultivation exercises, you can strengthen the center of the abdomen and retard the ineluctable flight of vital energy.

> The Tao is close, but everyone looks far away. Life is simple, but everyone seeks difficulty.
>
> —Men Tseu

3. OPENING THE SMALL CIRCULATION

The exercise of the small circulation provides an essential way of developing sexual potency through psychophysiological exercises that combine Taoist meditation, abdominal breathing, and the power of mind (visualization and mental imagery). The three treasures—*jing, qi,* and *shen*—are directly worked on in this exercise. A jade tablet dating from the sixth century B.C. describes the path taken by the energy flow during the meditation of the small circulation:

When one breathes in, energy descends. When energy descends, one becomes calm and energy becomes strong, whereupon it begins to germinate and then to push backward and rise up the back toward the crown of the head, and from there, it once again begins its descent.

Legend ascribes the invention of this traditional exercise to Lao-tzu himself, the founder of philosophical Taoism and master of the sexual exercises of the Yellow Chamber.

According to one story, a Taoist hermit who had practiced small-circulation meditation more than a hundred thousand times and used it during sexual intercourse was able to enter so completely into resonance with his partner that she found she could do the exercise herself with no effort at all and her own small circulation was activated as well.

This energy circuit also recalls other meditation practices, that of Indian tantric yoga in particular. Under the Tang dynasty, meditation was tied to sexual practices of yin-yang balance, and people spoke of a communication between the heart energies and the sexual organs. These methods, it was said, helped increase *jing*, that is, innate, or intrinsic, energy.

The Woman of Purity said:

If a man can practice the small circulation for three years, his *dantian* will be so powerful that he will achieve extraordinary physical strength; he will be able to keep an erection for a long time during sex.

THE BREATHING

Most of the errors that occur in the practice of small circulation come from improper breathing. Breathing during this exercise can be done in various ways with different rhythms: it should be light or forced; it should have a rapid or slow rhythm; it should be shallow or deep. The Taoist text known as the *Tao Tsang* speaks of a particular way of breathing: "Inhalation is continuous, exhalation is thin and drawn out."

YOUR INTERNAL ATTITUDE

According to tradition, the following three things are required of your internal attitude: your heart (your affective nature, your emotions) must be at peace; your determination must guide your *qi*; your *qi* must follow the movements of your breathing. For this, you will need to concentrate. The process is called *Hu Xi Dao Yin*, Guiding the Breath.

THE YIN CHANNEL AND THE YANG CHANNEL

These two channels form an energy circuit that begins at the perineum, passes up the back to the crown of the head, and then returns along the front of the body, passing through the *dantian* and the sexual organs. Taoists believe that anyone who wants to take the path of return toward original being must open these channels.

Practicing the small circulation will usually produce heat

sensations or pleasant vibrations throughout the abdomen and the genital organs and toward the sacrum, but these feelings should not be provoked consciously or sought out for their own sake. The practitioner should instead regard them with a certain objectivity and simply observe them as they occur.

THE METHOD FOR OPENING THE "SMALL CELESTIAL REVOLUTION"

The goal of this meditation is to make *qi* circulate toward the *Du* and *Ren* channels in order to create a lasting balance of yin and yang energies at every level of your being. Frequent circulation of an uninterrupted energy flow by means of this exercise will lead to better health, improved sexuality, and greater longevity. This meditation is practiced in a sitting position, either on a chair with your feet some distance apart or in a cross-legged or half-lotus position on the floor.

Begin the exercise in an attitude of calm and quietude. Cast aside all outside and chaotic thoughts and let your emotions be at peace. Then close your eyes gently, without forcing them shut, so that you allow a little light to pass beneath the lids; your jaws should be relaxed as you breathe lightly, gently, calmly, and continuously (in other words, at no time should there be any stoppage of the breath). Don't try to hold your breath, as is sometimes done in yoga. Your tongue should touch the roof of your mouth, thereby linking the *Du* and *Ren* channels at the *yinjiao* point, "the bridge of the feet."

You can hold your hands in one of two ways: the first

and simplest way is to let them rest on your kneecaps; the second way is to place one hand on top of the other, with both palms facing upward. This is the preferred position in Chan (the precursor of Zen). The thumbs should be touching each other.

After being in this position for a few moments, you should begin to feel a warm energy current appearing in the lower cinnabar field (*xia dantian*); this is the first stage. In men, this energy is yang; in women, it is yin.

Breathe through your nose (gently enough so that you are not making noise as you breathe in and out) as you slightly contract your anus upward and mentally guide *qi* along a trajectory from the *dantian* through the perineum, the sacrum, the lumbar, dorsal, and cervical vertebrae, and finally to the *Ba Hui* point at the crown of the head.

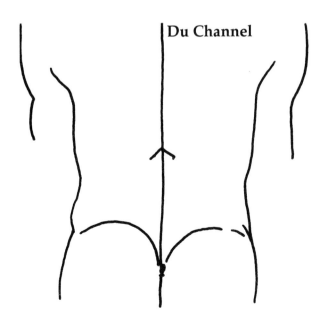

Du Channel

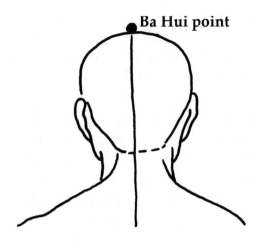

Ba Hui point

This entire trajectory is accomplished in one inhalation and should follow the pace of your breathing.

Then exhale through your nose—again, without making noise as you breath—while visualizing the descent of *qi* down the front of your body along the *Ren* channel as it makes its downward trajectory from the *Ba Hui* point through the lateral edges of each eye, the base of the tongue (the upper "bridge of the feet"),

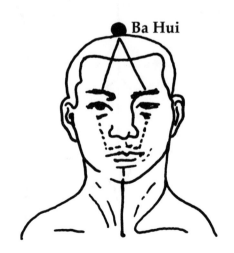

Ba Hui

then, as though you were swallowing *qi*, down the throat and the front of the chest to the lower cinnabar field and then back down toward the perineum. Throughout your exhalation, your stomach should protrude slightly forward.

In this way, an uninterrupted circuit is established:

Above and below, yin and yang rise and fall again and again; the fluid of life (*jing*) circulates ceaselessly in a circle; the purple palace and the limpid dragon (yin) communicate with the white tiger (yang); the mysterious palace (the pineal gland) and the axis of the earth (the *dantian*) join with the light of heaven (*qi*).

Throughout this exercise, your breathing should be slow and gentle (effortless), precise (with keen awareness), and regular (your inhalations should last as long as your exhalations, and there should be no stoppage of breath between these two phases, which should succeed one another naturally). In short, your breathing should be natural and unimpeded.

One of the greatest difficulties people encounter in performing this meditation consists of getting over what the ancients called "the three passes." These three stages are energy obstructions that result directly from the structure of the human anatomy: The first pass is located at the coccyx. The second is the *mingmen* point between the kidneys. The third is the "pillar of jade" at the occiput. These three passes are areas where it is difficult to feel *qi* as it flows past.

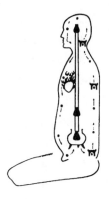

The small circulation.

Even if one does not believe that breath and air can travel throughout the body, there is no denying that *qi* travels in a very real sense along the imaginary trajectory, producing actual physiological and sensorial changes. This double nature of *qi* should make us reflect on the hypothesis that our body, as an energy field, has a profound relationship with our mind. Certain scientists today have no qualms about hypothesizing consciousness as the master of the physical universe. Might not the small circulation actually be an energy movement that imitates microcosmically the vast movements of the stars, thereby accelerating the process of human evolution?

Taoist theory speaks of the three precious pills of human life and sexual symbology: the celestial pill, which is the pure breaths that, in the process of normal abdominal or reverse breathing, reach down to the sexual centers; the terrestrial pill, comprising not only our earthly sustenance—what we eat and drink—but also the telluric energies; and the human pill, symbolizing one's sexual partner and his or her energies.

The small celestial circulation brings into play the three Taoist alchemical elements—wind, fire, and internal elixir: wind symbolizes breath and *qi*; fire symbolizes mental strength and concentration; and internal elixir symbolizes pure yang energy in a man and pure yin energy in a woman.

4. RESTORING SPRINGTIME

The two traditional Taoist exercises that follow were popularized in China by the internal schools and Bian Zhizhong, following the tradition of the Taoists of the Hua Shan mountains.

- One of the most important points in this exercise is the position of the spinal column: it must be perfectly straight but not rigid. Your back must be strong and supple; any stiffness will impede the flow of *qi*, thus diminishing the effects of the exercise and preventing energy from circulating as it should.

- Your shoulders should be relaxed, neither raised nor hunched over. This is not always easy to achieve, especially while you are learning the movements. The common tendency is to tense the shoulders, to raise them toward the neck and tuck the head into the shoulders.

- Hold your head straight, with your chin slightly tucked and your neck supple. The point on the top of the head between your two ears, on the line going from the nose to the nape of the neck, should be kept pointed toward the sky. Be careful not to lean your head forward or backward.

- Look straight ahead, neither to the right nor to the left (except as indicated for certain poses, in which, for example, you will need to follow the movements of your hands).

- Your hands should remain supple and elastic. When you close your fists, do so without exerting physical force. Don't clench them. If energy is circulating as it should, you will nonetheless feel as though there is great strength in your hands or your fingers, and an outside observer looking at your fists might imagine that they are being deliberately clenched with great force. This sign indicates that the energy is circulating.

- Your legs should remain supple as well. Do not tense them.

- The mobility and flexibility of your waist are very important. The waist is an axis, and from this axis the pelvis will move.

- Be persevering in your practice. Only through repetition will you obtain noticeable results.

- Learn to control your gaze: the eyes are the mirror of the mind; if you can master your eyes, you can master your mind.

- Practice this meditation at the same time every day in a quiet room kept at a pleasant temperature. It can also be practiced out of doors, in a place sheltered from wind, cold, sun, and damp.

- Let your breathing happen freely, and if you begin to feel short of breath, don't hesitate to breathe through your mouth, even if this goes against practices you may already be familiar with from other disciplines such as yoga.

- Don't let your mind stray or gravitate toward your everyday cares and worries. Remain wakeful and attentive, for this is also part of the exercise.
- Perform this movement without unnecessary effort, or mental tension. Of course, this is difficult to accomplish at first, but with daily practice you will master it.

This valuable exercise was still being practiced at the beginning of the century by the Taoist monks of the Hua mountains. It is practiced today in Taiwan and China. A most powerful exercise, it is capable of restoring lost vitality; it is also called "fortifying and nourishing the kidneys and breath."

As you know by now, the word "kidney" should be understood here in a broad sense, that is, as vitality, longevity, sexual force, and reproduction. For the ancient Taoists all these notions resided in this simple word.

The following exercise and the one preceding it should be practiced regularly, twice a day for at least three minutes. This exercise stimulates the circulation of *qi* and blood, of yin and yang; increases vitality through the influx of fresh, pure *qi*; expels stagnant, used *qi*; stimulates the five viscera, particularly the kidneys, and the sexual organs (when practiced with the exercise that comes after it); and normalizes body weight.

With its simple three-part movement, this exercise should be practiced in a natural and supple way; you should never force your breathing. Here is how it is traditionally done.

PREPARATION

Stand with your feet shoulder-width apart from each other. Relax the muscles in your arms, letting your hands rest alongside your thighs. Keep your knees slightly bent. Look straight ahead of you, focusing into infinity. Keep your eyes half open, your gaze tranquil. Empty your mind of all its cares and thoughts.

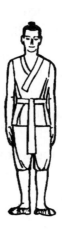

FIRST PART: INHALING VITALIZING QI

Inhale as you lift your heels gently off the floor, without losing your balance.

Visualize the fresh air penetrating everywhere inside you, stimulating every cell of your body.

Gradually shift your weight onto the balls and toes of your feet, without forcing your breathing or making noise as you breathe. Then exhale while lowering your heels gently to the floor, ending with a slight bend in the knees. Do this on a single exhalation, letting your back curve outward just a bit and your stomach cave in slightly.

As the air leaves your lungs, visualize it carrying all your toxins away with it.

Perform this first part sixteen times in succession, slowly, but breathing completely.

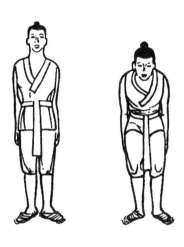

SECOND PART: SHAKING THE BODY AND CHASING OUT THE TOXINS

Check to see that your knees are still bent, and then relax.

Breathe naturally as you shake your entire body with a series of harmonious vibrations to a rapid rhythm (three vibrations a second, if possible). Do this for about a minute, while breathing freely.

You might be a bit surprised at first, and you should not force the movement; little by little, as you relax more and more, you will begin to feel the vibrations shake your body (as this happens, try to keep your shoulders, jaws, and pelvis relaxed).

Men will feel their testicles swinging to a rapid rhythm, and women will feel their breasts jump and their vagina relax.

If you find it difficult to get the vibration going, try shaking your body from top to bottom and from front to back slightly. With practice, the vibration will come naturally.

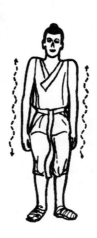

THIRD PART: RELAXING YOUR INTERNAL ORGANS

Gently bend your right knee and rotate your right shoulder forward and downward toward the middle of the body (see figure on next page.), and then upward and outward in a smooth, harmonious circle. Now do the same with your left shoulder as you bend your left knee. This movement will soon become natural. Do not force the movement of your shoulders.

Breathe naturally as you perform this exercise sixteen times.

Little by little, you will feel the yin-yang movement of your waist, as one side opens outward and the other closes inward. You will also feel a definite effect on the stomach.

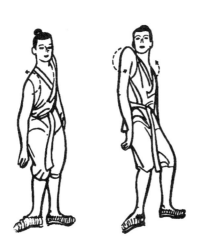

5. FORTIFYING THE SEXUAL ORGANS

This exercise is unique in that it fortifies the sexual organs in both men and women. It is said that the courtesans of the last emperors of China, anxious to reap the benefits of this exercise, would make the journey to the Hua mountains just to learn it. With its tonic effect on the male and female sexual organs, this exercise acts directly on the kidneys, the adrenal glands, the sexual glands, and the pelvis and on many acupuncture points and channels as well. This exercise is said to strengthen kidney functioning, relieve lumbago, firm and lift the vagina, and stimulate blood flow in the testicles (which can prevent varicoceles and genital inflammations).

Practiced on a regular basis, this exercise can also help prevent nocturnal emissions and involuntary seminal emissions in young men. And like the previous exercise, it increases the tone of the breasts in young women.

PREPARATION

Take the same position as in the previous exercise, with your back straight but relaxed.

THE MOVEMENT

Raise your left hand slowly, keeping your palm upward in front of the body, until your hand reaches the height of your chest. At the same time, describe an arc with the right foot and set it down to the right, as indicated in the figure on the next page.

Then raise your right hand to the level of your lower ribs, as you bring your left hand in front of your face, holding it as though it were a mirror (keep your left elbow bent, as in the figure). At the same time, pivot your left foot on the toe, moving your heel in an outward direction; then squeeze your buttocks as hard as you can, pressing them together so that you can feel your genital organs.

Repeat these movements from the other side.

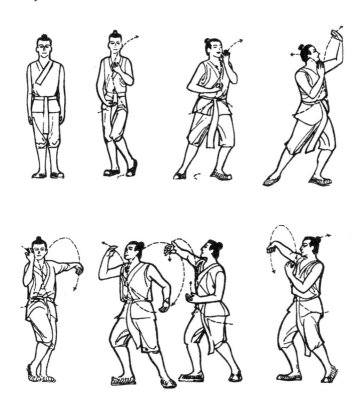

Do this exercise eight times on each side. Be sure to perform the movements slowly, keeping your breathing relaxed and unforced throughout. (Women should never perform this exercise during their periods or during pregnancy.)

6. FORTIFYING THE KIDNEYS

This ancient exercise stimulates what the Taoists call the cinnabar field, the energy point in the middle of the abdomen, which connects a person's vital reserves (linked to the kidneys and *jing,* or vital and sexual essence) with his or her *qi,* or readily available force.

Traces of this exercise can be found in a seventeenth-century Taoist compilation that speaks of the exercises of the immortals. The "immortals" were Taoist sages and hermits who, having realized their energy potential, attained a high degree of spiritual accomplishment. The *daoyin* exercise is simply called "holding your feet."

Sit down on the floor with your legs tensed and grasp the soles of your feet, with your hands reaching around the outside of the foot to the sole.

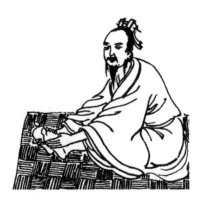

Remain in this position as you take nine deep breaths, keeping your awareness focused on the abdomen. Don't force your breathing; you can keep your eyes halfway closed to help you concentrate.

7. MASSAGING THE THREE SEXUAL ENERGY GATES

This acupressure massage of the energy points is good for both sexes; it can help both men and women prolong the sex act and increase their orgasmic pleasure.

This massage uses the same pressure-and-release method described in the section on the female aphrodisiac acupressure point: press the points with the thumb until you begin to feel discomfort, then release without lifting your thumb from the skin; repeat this cycle of pressure and release for about two minutes on each of the three energy gates, in the following order.

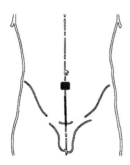

First point.

The first point is located two centimeters below the navel. You can feel it by pressing gently with the index finger on the skin; you will feel a slight depression there.

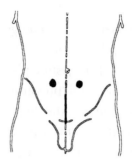

Second point.

The second point (there are actually two of them) is located three centimeters below the navel, four centimeters to either side of the midline.

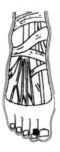

Third point.

The third point is located at the base of the nail of the second toe, toward the outside of the toe.

These three massages should be repeated once a day for three weeks.

8. *NEIYANG GONG*: INTERNAL STRENGTHENING

Neiyang gong is a mental relaxation method for sexual opening. We have already seen some of the many subtle ways in which thoughts of inadequacy and emotional upset can give rise to sexual inhibitions in men and women. These inhibitions, if not addressed, will eventually worsen and become permanent energy disorders; that is why all the preceding exercises are advised for those who suffer from impotence or frigidity. Taoist meditation practices are another useful remedy, especially when these conditions result from emotional or psychological causes. These practices can help the sufferer free himself or herself from the obsessional thoughts that can dim the mind as clouds hide the sun.

Obsessional thoughts can afflict anyone, not just people with clinically diagnosed emotional disorders; all of us at one time or another have found ourselves swept into the cycle of conflictual emotions: anger (it's always justified, isn't it?), passions (they're pleasant at first, but, as we all know, they soon turn destructive), supreme joy (if one's wedding is the happiest day of one's life, how can the remainder of one's life be anything but grim?), grief (he left me, I didn't deserve that! We *have* to suffer, it's karma), and so on.

Taoist therapy considers different agents or conditions to be potential sources of mental disorders. Impotence, for example, is linked to excessive worries, frustration, melancholy, and fear, as well as to physical or energy problems such as kidney deficiencies or digestive troubles. Taoist medicine draws no borders between physical and emotional causes, which simply goes to show that Chinese therapists were well ahead of their time in grasping the concept of psychosomatic illness.

Even the six pathogenic atmospheric influences—wind, cold, heat, dampness, dryness, and fire—were considered factors that could aggravate the emotions. For extreme emotional disturbances, in particular the yang-type disorders such as rage, epilepsy, and manias, Taoist physicians prescribed fasting to reduce *qi*, which exacerbates these conditions. It was even said that extreme weather conditions on the day of conception could trigger irreversible mental troubles in the newborn child: an excess of yin could produce retardation; a child conceived during a heat wave would turn out to be hot tempered. For example, the phrase in Taoist therapy corresponding to the Western word *depression* is "stagnation of *qi*, accompanied by deficiency of *qi*," according to texts from the Ming dynasty period (1368–1644).

The best therapy for disorders that are emotional in origin or manifestation is, beyond a doubt, Taoist meditation, the internal healing method of *neiyang gong*. This method, part of the *qigong* discipline, had been transmitted orally from master to disciple until 1947, when Dr. Liu Gui Zhen asked Liu Du Zhou, the great *qigong* master from the province of Hebei, to reveal the method publicly for the sake of sick people everywhere. Dr. Liu simplified the meditation and adapted it to the needs and capabilities of his hospital patients. Internal healing quickly proved its effectiveness in producing therapeutic results. Its reputation soon spread throughout China, and it is now practiced and taught in the largest hospitals of traditional Chinese medicine, especially in Shanghai.

Neiyang gong has a calming effect on brain activity, while amplifying the vital functions. Additionally, the basis of this technique—the repetition of a phrase—helps increase mental tranquility through positive suggestion. The main sexual indications for the use of this method include impotence, spermatorrhea, prostatitis, genital infections, premature ejaculation, inflammation of the uterus, dysmenorrhea, and prolapse of the uterus. The list, longer today than it was in the 1950s, owes its expansion to successful outcomes in many clinical trials.

GENERAL SUGGESTIONS FOR PRACTICING NEIYANG GONG

Before each breathing exercise and each concentration exercise, you should disengage yourself from all your preoccupations. Your breathing should be slow and relaxed. If you are not sufficiently calm while performing this exercise, do not insist on continuing it. It is better to do something else.

Whether you are performing this exercise in a sitting or reclining position, you should wear loose clothing that does not impede your breathing or restrict blood circulation (belts, buckles, and constricting undergarments can be particularly problematic—it's best not to wear them). Your breathing should not be tense or forced, and you should be able to relax the muscles of your entire body. Your gaze should fall naturally down your nose or to your toes, and your eyes should be half closed. If your eyes are tired, however, feel free to close them, unless this puts you to sleep. In that case, it is better to keep them slightly open.

The position of your body during this exercise should be

natural, loose, and unconstrained. Whichever position you take—sitting, reclining, or standing—be sure not to thrust your chest forward or tense your shoulders: maintaining the pose should require no effort. If you choose to sit, it is recommended that, once you have assumed this position, you try leaning your upper body slightly forward, backward, to the right, and to the left, until you find the position that is ideal for you.

People using this meditation technique to treat a chronic illness or people with severe illness should practice sexual abstinence for one hundred days and eat simple, light meals. This period of sexual abstinence should begin at the start of this cure; if the hoped-for improvements do not occur, the period of abstinence should be extended.

NEIYANG GONG: INTERNAL HEALING EXERCISE

Here is a complete description of this health-promoting exercise in which a person, sitting or lying down, transforms his shallow breathing into breathing that is calm and long. Its benefits are enhanced through the mental repetition of certain syllables.

There are three basic positions for practicing internal healing. The position you choose will depend on personal taste or circumstance. For example, a fatigued, hospitalized, or otherwise bedridden person would probably opt for one of the two reclining positions.

First position: Lying on your side. To maintain proper posture during the exercise, make sure that the bed is not too soft. If you are cold, you can cover yourself with a blanket.

It doesn't matter on which side you lie, unless you have just eaten, in which case you should lie on your right side: in that position the stomach is less heavy. You can bend your arm if you like and rest your forearm on a cushion, palm facing outward, your hand three thumb widths (about six centimeters) from your head. If you are lying on your right side, place your left hand lightly on your thigh, palm facing downward. Keep the leg that is in contact with the mattress extended and slightly tensed; the other leg should be bent at about a 120-degree angle. Then lay your bent leg on top of the other leg. With your eyes half closed, your gaze should now rest on your nose or your toes. Keep your mouth closed.

Second position: Sitting. This exercise is performed on a chair or stool. The soles of your feet should be touching the floor. Your knees should be bent at a ninety-degree angle. Your bearing should be stable. Your chest should incline neither forward nor backward, neither to the right nor to the left. Rest your hands on your thighs and spread your legs so that your feet are shoulder-width apart. Your eyes should be open only a slit while you let your gaze rest on your nose or your toes.

Third position: Lying on your back. Lie down on your bed, without contracting your muscles. The bed should be hard, and your cushion should be placed higher than for the first position (two palm widths). Support your shoulders with a cushion about four thumb widths (eight centimeters) in thickness. Here, too, your eyes should be open no more than a slit, and you should be looking down at your nose or your toes.

Once you have assumed the proper position, begin

breathing through your nose. Breathe normally at first for one or two minutes, then begin silently repeating the syllables indicated below. As you inhale, the tip of your tongue should touch the palate and remain there for a brief instant; as you exhale, let your tongue fall back down to the floor of the mouth. Repeat these breathing movements at a regular pace as you say the syllables to yourself.

To begin with, say in your mind a three-syllable word or phrase, for example, "I am calm." Of course, you should really *be* calm in this case. If you like, you can say other words, such as "one, two, three."

Progressively increase the number of syllables, but only after a week or two of practice with three syllables. Always breathe in on the first syllable, hold your breath on the second, and exhale only on the last syllable. You can increase the number of syllables in multiples of three. The interval during which you hold your breath will become longer and longer but should never exceed three syllables, as you inhale for the first three syllables, hold your breath for the next three, and exhale for the last three. For example: "my spirit" (inhalation) "is at rest" (retention of breath) "without thoughts" (exhalation).

How long you extend this interval is up to you: it is for you to decide how long each cycle should last. But in any case the cycle will have three phases: inhalation, retention, exhalation. There is no intervening phase between your exhalation and your inhalation; inhalation should immediately follow exhalation. You should breathe naturally and at a regular pace; there should be no feeling of suffocation or respiratory distress (dyspnea). This way of breathing is called "normal" breathing; there are other ways of breathing that will be described later.

In the beginning, it can be rather difficult to attain a state of perfect concentration. What we mean here by concentration is not mental effort directed toward a particular point, but rather an absence of the disruptive thoughts that come with sensory awareness. To achieve this concentration as you perform the exercise, focus—without forcing yourself—on the *dantian*, located about two thumb widths below the navel. After about twenty days of daily practice, you will begin to feel as though your breath is reaching all the way down to your abdominal cavity, as though the air is descending into your belly. Later you will be able to generalize this sensation and feel it anywhere in your body, as part of the Taoist self-healing process.

The exercise described above is a concentration exercise: by concentrating on the *dantian*—the abdominal energy center or cinnabar field—you will eventually attain the state of total calm called *rujing*.

This focus is difficult to achieve at first. Beginners can usually concentrate only for a short time before their thoughts begin to stray. This is to be expected. While you are "preserving your *dantian*," as the Chinese would say, you should not attempt to force yourself to concentrate. Since the *dantian* can be thought of as an "object" that lies halfway between the real and the imaginary, any inordinate effort on your part can provoke psychic overexertion and impede the progress of the meditation.

Those who are practicing this meditation for simple disease prevention, longevity, or sexual well-being should do it once or twice a day, at the same hour every day if possible. Ideally, internal healing should be practiced for thirty minutes to one hour in the morning and another thirty minutes in the evening before you go to bed. Beginners should start with periods of shorter duration (ten to fifteen minutes) so as not to cause psychic tension.

Those who wish to remedy a particular sexual problem should refer to the following table and choose their meditation program according to their specific needs:

PROBLEM	FREQUENCY	DURATION	RESPIRATION	CONCENTRATION
Impotence	Twice	10 to 30 minutes	Normal or Special 2	Abdomen
Spermatorrhea	Two to three times	10 to 30 minutes	Normal or Special 2	Abdomen
Genital infections	Two to three times	10 to 30 minutes	Normal or Special 2	Abdomen
Dysmenorrhea	Two to three times	10 to 30 minutes	Special 2	Abdomen
Prolapse of the uterus	Two to three times	10 to 30 minutes	Normal	Abdomen
Frigidity	Two to three times	10 to 30 minutes	Normal	Abdomen

9. TAPPING THE ESSENCE OF THE SUN AND THE NECTAR OF THE MOON

The *qigong* exercises for gathering the essence of the sun and the nectar of the moon are important methods used by ancient Taoists to tone yang and supplement yin and thereby increase the pure sexual energies associated with these two polarities. Taoists believed that these methods were sufficient in themselves to treat male impotence and female frigidity.

Sun essence can increase the body's yang energy, while

moon nectar tones yin essence and the normal body fluids. Yang represents vital energy that is immediately available to the body to defend itself physically and mentally, while yin is the body's sap or quintessence in the form of body fluids (of which hormones are one example).

VISUALIZATION EXERCISE FOR COLLECTING THE YANG ESSENCE OF THE SUN

The energy of the rising sun is yang-type energy; it polarizes the qi of the air, making it more vivifying and tonic. Taoists think that modern science has yet to grasp all the riches of our universe's subtle vibrations; the effect of sunspots and light rays and the flow of particles are examples of phenomena that are still not well understood. Taoists believe that exposure to rays of sunlight in the morning induces a healthy awakening of the vital forces. The five viscera all benefit from this flow of life, as do one's mental capacities.

This meditation tones the essential sexual energies in their pure yang aspect.

In preparation, stand facing the sun with your feet spread shoulder-width apart, knees slightly bent; remain in a state of relaxation and tranquility, breathe regularly, and rid yourself of all interfering or negative thoughts.

As the sun rises above the horizon, lower your eyelids slightly, keeping them open just enough so that you can perceive its reddish light (if the sun is hidden by clouds, simply imagine that you are seeing it rise); as you breathe in through the nose, inhale the qi essence of the solar light; breathe in a good mouthful of this essence (in your imagination, of course), and hold your breath for a moment as you focus your mind; then exhale, and as you do so, swallow this essence while sending puffs of it down to your *dantian* (the Elixir Field, located in the middle of the abdomen, below your navel). This process constitutes the first part of the exercise. Swallow this essence naturally, as though you were drinking water from a glass; with practice this will become natural and pleasant. At the completion of the exercise, swallow ten times.

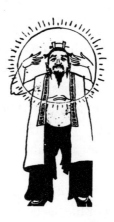

Absorbing the solar light.

Then relax naturally, let your mind concentrate peacefully for a brief instant, then stretch your limbs for a moment just as you would normally. This visualization exercise can also be practiced shortly after sunrise, in the early morning. For maximum intensity, however, performing it at actual sunrise is best.

VISUALIZATION EXERCISE FOR COLLECTING THE YIN NECTAR OF THE MOON

The moon represents the body's yin energies and fluids. In traditional Chinese medicine, the balance of sexual fluids is closely related to mental health and the ability to find inner peace. In Asia, intelligence and the ability to meditate are often represented symbolically by the moon. The moon is also related to the woman's menstrual cycle and its regular progression. The ancient Taoists said that if a woman practiced this exercise regularly, she would become more feminine and would have a luminous, glowing aura, perfect health, and stable mental energy. This exercise is not for women alone, however; men too can benefit from this simple practice, which will calm their yang if it is overly exuberant or impulsive. It's also a good way for men to calm nervous tensions and aggressive drives and to balance their hormonal system.

In preparation, find an open spot out of doors at night and stand facing the moon as you enter a state of relaxation and tranquility, breathing regularly and ridding yourself of all interfering thoughts. It is not advisable to perform this exercise completely naked.

Lower your eyelids until you can barely make out the moon; breathe in through your nose and mouth, gently inhaling the nectar of the moon as you take in a mouthful of this nectar (you should visualize this); hold your breath gently as you concentrate your mind and swallow the nectar slowly, sending it down to the abdominal *dantian* (the Elixir Field, in the middle of the belly, three thumb widths below the navel). This process constitutes the second part of the exercise. Repeat it six times. This meditation may seem a little abstract, but with practice, it will become easy and natural. Then you will really have the feeling of absorbing the nectar of the moon.

To finish, concentrate peacefully for a brief instant on the inner feeling of your body and mind, then stretch your limbs naturally.

This lunar meditation, when done in autumn and at full moon, is particularly good for the blood and for the feminine energies.

CHAPTER FOUR

Green Dragon and White Tiger:

The Sexual Union

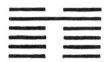

THE TREATISE of the Yellow Emperor sheds yet more light on the dyadic nature of sexual practice:

> The Yellow Emperor said to Su Nu: "I have understood the general concept of the interplay of yin and yang. Can you give me more details?"
>
> Su Nu answered: "All earthly creations depend on yin and yang. Birth is brought about by the union of yin and yang. Thus it is that when a man's penis is in contact with a woman, it becomes erect. When the woman is stimulated, her lips open. Thus yin and yang enter into contact. The sperm and the female fluids blend together."

THE NUMBERS SEVEN, EIGHT, NINE, AND TEN: TRADITIONAL TAOIST COUNSELS

THE SEVEN DANGERS

A book written on bamboo tablets was discovered in Mawangdui in 1974. In this book, titled *Tian Xia Zhi Dao Tan* (The Tao of the world), the Taoist author describes difficulties that can arise during sex and explains several methods for achieving balance within it.

The "Seven Dangers" and "Eight Methods" constitute the main part of the book. The former are things that a person must avoid to remain sexually potent, while the eight methods represent steps that can be taken to counter those threats and strengthen sexuality. This text is the first attempt in the history of Chinese medicine to treat the theme of human sexuality.

The seven dangers are:

1. Internal closure. During sex, the man feels a sudden pain in his penis, or his seminal duct closes, blocking the flow of sperm.
2. Outward emanation of alcohol. This condition, which manifests itself in profuse sweating during sexual relations, signals an excessive consumption of alcohol.
3. Exhaustion. Sexual intemperance diminishes the sperm (creating internal dryness) and weakens vital energy (*qi*).
4. Impotence. This condition is a sign of profound fatigue that needs to be corrected with yang tonics, blood tonics, or *qi* tonics.
5. Indifference. A lack of interest during sex can bring on shortness of breath and vertigo. It also tends to make sex a purely mechanical affair.
6. Female impasse. The penis penetrates too quickly and cannot satisfy the woman if she wants to achieve orgasm.
7. Flight of energy. The rapid loss of energy shortens the sex act.

These seven dangers are harmful for sexual harmony not only on the level of physical energies but also on the spiritual level. These dangers are taken up in somewhat different form in the *Su Nu Jing*, the classic work attributed to the Yellow Emperor, in which they are described as follows:

1. The drying up of secretions due to overstimulation.
2. Overly frequent ejaculation resulting in loss of *jing*.
3. Irregular pulse caused by sexual excitement that exceeds one's internal forces.
4. The loss of *qi* resulting from having sex while in a state of fatigue.
5. Internal dysfunction aggravated by having sex before one has completely recovered from an illness affecting one of the five internal organs.
6. The hundred difficulties that arise when the woman becomes so ravenous for sex that her hunger cannot be satisfied.
7. Hematuria, which occurs when a man who is already tired from his ordinary activities exhausts himself further by having sex without taking his reserves into account. He can seriously weaken his kidneys and begin to urinate blood.

THE EIGHT METHODS

The eight methods are internal exercises that are to be practiced along with breathing exercises. Through a process of relaxation and harmonization, these methods make it possible to achieve true sexual harmony.

They are as follows:

1. Good breath circulation (*qi*). Sit with your legs folded, back straight, buttocks relaxed, and anus slightly contracted upward; then direct your *qi* toward the lower abdomen, until it reaches your sexual organs.

2. Releasing the first secretions. Stand with your legs shoulder-width apart, bend your legs at the knee, as in the mounted archer's pose described earlier. Breathe deeply into the abdominal region, move your tongue around in your mouth, then swallow your saliva and relax your buttock muscles. Direct your *qi* downward to the sex organs, holding your back straight and keeping your anus gently contracted so that the sexual organs release the first lubricating secretions.

3. Seizing the moment. The partners caress each other's body and engage in sexual foreplay. Then they relax physically and mentally before having sexual intercourse. Sexual intercourse begins only when the desire for it appears.

4. Accumulating *qi*. At the moment the sex act begins, with your back relaxed and anus slightly contracted, make your *qi* descend so that it concentrates in your sexual organs.

5. Stimulating the release of the sweet secretion. The penis penetrates gently, slowly, and harmoniously to encourage the release of secretions from the genital organs.

6. Conserving *qi*. Draw out the penis while it is still rigid, before ejaculation occurs.

7. Conserving *qi* until climax. As sexual intercourse is

about to reach conclusion, stop moving and circulate your *qi* up and down the spinal column, then make it descend so that you accumulate as much energy as possible in the *dantian*.

8. Pouring out the waters of *jing*. This means that ejaculation takes place outside the vagina.

In the Mawangdui treatise, the eight methods are said to be good for the energies of both partners and thus promote conjugal harmony. According to this text,

> Whoever practices the eight methods and avoids the seven dangers will have keen hearing, sharp vision, and a svelte and supple body; he will enjoy good health and will live to a ripe old age.

THE NINE ENERGIES

The *Su Nu Jing* also describes the nine energies or principles that can help prevent a sexual relationship from becoming a source of illness and keep pleasure from turning into pain. In some ways, these principles recall the Western concept of the golden mean:

> During the sex act, human beings are subject to the nine energies.
> If these energies are not heeded, the man's body will be afflicted with ulcers, inflammations, and edema, and the woman will suffer from irregular periods and other maladies.
> Total disregard of these rules can even cause death,

but if the man and the woman obey the principles of yin and yang, they will enjoy good health, joy, and long life. This then is the principle of the sex act. It is a principle of mental stability, emotional balance, harmonious energy, and physical and mental fitness.

One should avoid extremes in life: One should expose oneself neither to extreme cold nor to extreme heat; one should neither fast nor gorge. One should maintain a perfect moral and physical code of ethics and always seek peace both within oneself and with others.

THE TEN PRECIOUS RECOMMENDATIONS

Zhang Jiebin, author of another classic Chinese treatise, set down these ten counsels:

1. Choose the right moment for conception. There are biorhythms that make it possible to have sex when the conditions that favor conception come together.
2. The partners' search for simultaneous orgasm can allow both the man and the woman to achieve complete satisfaction through the interaction of their yin and yang energies.
3. The sexuality of spouses will differ according to their respective physical constitutions. If the man is in better health than his wife, he should do all he can to surround her with care and attention before they make love. If, on the other hand, the woman is in better health than the man, she should be patient and wait until his penis is hard.

4. Insufficient accumulation of *qi* is at the origin of erectile dysfunction; therefore, *qi* must be nourished by every means possible.

5. The daily accumulation of sperm is just as important as its emission. If the man neglects either one, he risks ruining his health.

6. Moderation must be practiced in sexual relations: a person must be well rested before having sex and not make love when very tired; one must exercise restraint in sexual relations and not have sex too often.

7. Good humor is an important condition for ensuring a happy and lasting sex life.

8. Having sex during the last months of pregnancy is inadvisable because of the risk of provoking a spontaneous abortion.

9. Old persons and the infirm should absolutely avoid conception.

10. Sexual desire results from natural drives and originates in the body's internal organs, in other words, when *jing* and *qi* of the kidneys are strong. Any desire that springs purely from fantasies will harm the quality of sexual relations.

THE GREAT TAOIST PRINCIPLES OF NATURAL SEX

THE AGES OF LOVE

Sun Si-miao, the physician of the Tang dynasty period known for both his medical expertise and his great virtue, lived for over a hundred years. A specialist in sexology, he devoted a chapter of his book, *Precious Prescriptions for*

Emergency Cases, to this subject. In this treatise he emphasized two critical periods in a man's sexual life: A man of forty years needs to be particularly aware of the relation between energy and sexual activity. Practicing the pleasures of the flesh as he did in his youth will have grave consequences for his physical and mental health. For this reason, a man should retain his sperm during the sex act; in other words, he should be careful not to emit his sperm too frequently. If he does not observe these precautions, he will weaken physically or age prematurely; he can even drop dead when all his sperm has been depleted. As for young men, even if they enjoy an iron constitution, they should not indulge in sexual pleasures too early in life or indulge in masturbation, for these things will make them lose their *jing* prematurely.

The *Xuan Nu Jing* speaks to this same subject:

If a man tries to have orgasm too often, he will gravely damage his health. He must adhere to the following frequencies of ejaculation [this advice concerns only ejaculatory frequency, not the frequency of sexual relations]:

A young man of fifteen years in perfect health can ejaculate twice a day; if he is tired, only once a day.

A twenty-year-old man can ejaculate twice a day.

A thirty-year-old man can ejaculate once a day; once every two days if he is tired.

A forty-year-old man can ejaculate once every three days.

A fifty-year-old man can ejaculate once every five days; if he is sick, once every ten days.

A sixty-year-old man can ejaculate once every ten days; once every twenty days if he is sick.

A seventy-year-old man can ejaculate once a month, but if he is sick, he should refrain from ejaculating altogether.

MODERATION

On the subject of moderation, the *Xuan Nu Jing* states:

Lack of moderation in sexual relations can provoke abcesses in men and gynecological ailments in women; through immoderation, both men and women risk diminishing their longevity. Those who know how to husband their energies are happy and robust and will live to be old.

CONJUGAL HARMONY

On the subject of conjugal harmony, the *Xuan Nu Jing* states:

At the moment of the sex act, if the woman has no desire and does not secrete vaginal fluids, can the man have a stiff and potent penis?

Xuan Nu answered: "A happy and harmonious sex life depends on conjugal harmony. If one of the partners lacks desire, the sexual hormones will not elicit secretions from either partner. In that case, it is useless to talk of pleasure."

THE OCCASIONAL AVOIDANCE OF EJACULATION

The woman of Glory asked, "Isn't the goal of sexual intercourse to obtain pleasure through ejaculation? If one refrains from ejaculating, what point is there in having sex?" The Taoist master answered: "Usually, after ejaculation, the man feels tired and sleepy; sometimes he is thirsty and his ears ring. Although he recovers rather quickly from these conditions, they can hardly be called agreeable. By avoiding ejaculation from time to time, the man will increase his energy, improve his eyesight, and sharpen his hearing. Additionally, by refraining from ejaculating he will increase his sexual energy and be able to have sex more often, which is a better reward than momentary ejaculatory pleasure."

VIOLENT WEATHER CONDITIONS

Sexual relations should be avoided during extreme weather conditions such as heat waves, severe cold, storms, eclipses, floods, and thunderstorms; at such times, the yin and yang magnetic energies of the earth are in a state of upheaval, and human energy is sensitive to these atmospheric conditions.

VIOLENT EMOTIONS

Avoid sexual relations during periods of emotional upset— rage, grief, after a great fright, if you are intoxicated with drugs or alcohol, or after overeating. Sexual intercourse, as we have seen, sets into play energies of the profoundest sort. Since violent emotional conditions are extremely disruptive of internal yang *qi* energy, these conditions can increase the sexual energies and even make them permanent. The ancient texts warn against having sexual relations under such conditions, which can "produce illness in men and women or cause a stillbirth, if the union happens to be fruitful and leads to conception."

ILLNESSES

Avoid having sexual relations if one of the two partners has a serious chronic illness. Sexual union under such conditions will tire both partners. Sexual intercourse during or immediately after a "hot" illness (especially fevers) can cause serious complications and hinder recovery. The seriously ill should abstain from sex in order to conserve their *jing* and strengthen their body's immune system. Some may find this hard, but it is sometimes the only way to recovery.

THE PHASES OF THE MOON

Having sexual relations on the first day of the lunar cycle (on the new moon) is unfavorable, particularly for the energies of the mind. The reason for this rule has to do with principles of Taoist bioenergetics, which are too involved to enter into here.

THE ANAL ORIFICE

Avoid having sexual relations via the anal orifice. The Taoist texts are explicit on this point and maintain that anal sex (including anal sex in a homosexual relationship) seriously inverts the yin and yang energies and is at the root of many exogenous disorders.

MENSTRUAL PERIODS

Having sexual relations during menstruation "brings illness to both women and men."

MASTURBATION

Masturbation entails a great loss of energy (seminal essence) if practiced too frequently. Moreover, Taoists consider it dangerous to "make love with phantoms." Masturbating hinders the attainment of the emptiness of mind that facilitates meditation and mental relaxation. From adolescence until age twenty, it is not good to rush headlong into sexual adventures or masturbation. At this age, a person's *jing*, or sexual essence, is still somewhat weak, and self-abuse during this period will have disastrous results later in life and will ultimately diminish the strength of the organism's immune system.

SEXUAL ENERGY AND THE INTERNAL ORGANS

When vital energy is excited, it reaches the liver, and the penis, now aroused, becomes erect; when vital energy reaches the heart, the swollen penis feels some of this heat; when vital energy arrives at the kidneys, the penis becomes rigid and powerful.

THE FIVE FEMALE REACTIONS

As for the woman, she should have five reactions: when *qi* reaches her heart, her face reddens; when it reaches her liver, she looks everywhere around her—a sign of love; when *qi* reaches her lungs, she says not another word and her nose becomes moist; when it reaches her spleen, she nestles her neck against her partner's; when it reaches her kidneys, her vagina opens and lubricates.

DELICATE MOMENTS

The classic medical texts also advise against sexual relations at specific times that correspond to moments of shift in yin and yang energies: at noon, at midnight, during a solar eclipse, during a lunar eclipse, when there is a rainbow, at the summer and winter solstices, at full moon, and on a full stomach.

Since the energy of the human body is a microcosm contained within a vast macrocosm that surrounds it, such periods of high polarization can engender an energy imbalance in the physical and mental constitution of a child who is conceived at such times. Chinese medicine, like Chinese culture in general, is based on principles of moderation. All extremes are considered potentially dangerous. For example, a child conceived during one of these periods will tend to be special and "not like other children."

THE MOURNING PERIOD

Conceiving a child during times of grief is ill-advised because of the energy relation between *shen* and *jing* (kidney essence), the source of the sexual energies and body fluids. Severe mental depression can also affect the quality of procreative energy.

SEXUAL ABSTINENCE

There is no getting around the fact that in the past many Taoist masters have counseled and preached sexual abstinence. Now that you have grasped the importance of *jing* in the process of spiritual development, you also understand that any loss of *jing* represents a diminishment not only of vitality but also of intellectual faculties and concentration. Other masters have gone even further, maintaining that sexual thoughts of any sort, in men and women alike, also constitute a loss of *jing*. It is clear, however, that the restraint they advocate is impossible for most human beings. Therefore, most Taoists take a more moderate position.

After the age of twenty, the wisest thing to do, Taoists believe, is have sex about once a week. Certain teachings maintain that only those sex acts in which sperm is emitted should count; we believe that this is false, however, since any sexual stimulation represents a loss of *jing*. It makes no difference whether this stimulation involves sexual intercourse, masturbation, or mere arousal without ejaculation or orgasm: sexuality constitutes a deployment of the body's deepest energies. As Sun Si-miao has shown, as one advances in years and one's capacities decline, one's sex life should taper off as well; people over seventy-five, he advised, should not have sex at all, so that they can preserve their energies.

THE SEX ACT

SHOULD EJACULATION BE HELD BACK?

A number of books have come out in the West that speak of the possibility of ejaculatory retention through various mental, energetic, or even physical means, such as blocking the seminal ducts with the application of pressure on the central point of the perineum. These methods are in no way sanctioned by all Taoist schools, and in those schools where they are practiced they are always carried out under the authority and supervision of an experienced master. These methods are dangerous and can bring considerable frustration at first and energy troubles later.

Most of these practices have their origin in a misreading

of an ancient Taoist text, the essentials of which we cite here:

> When a man feels that he is going to ejaculate, he should close his mouth and open his eyes wide.
>
> Above all he should try to harmonize his breathing and hold his breath if he can, but without forcing the air into his chest. By moving his hands up and down and by breathing only from the lower abdomen, he can control his breath and his semen. During this sexual practice he should keep his spine straight.
>
> If necessary, he can press with the index finger and third finger of his left hand against acupuncture point Ping I (a thumb width above the nipple of the right breast) and then exhale through his nose, while pressing his jaws together.
>
> This is the method for holding back the sperm so that it can rise unimpeded and nourish the brain. If the man lets his sperm escape outside of him, he will damage his spirit *(shen)*.

This text does not seem to suggest that this method be practiced on a regular basis. Moreover, Taoists know that unreleased energy remains in the belly and stagnates there. There are ways, of course, to direct this energy toward the brain in order to rejuvenate it—the small-circulation method, the basics of which are described above, is one way—but even then, this energy can provoke congestions in the head. Sexual force, if restrained, is like dynamite! It can be used positively or negatively, and only a spiritual master can help you release yourself from the internal pressure of this energy. Taoists follow the natural course: ejaculation and orgasm are natural, whereas seminal retention is an artificial act that affects both the mind and the physical energies. Taoists refer to unemitted sperm as "dead jing."

This dead *jing*, moreover, can accumulate in the prostate gland and produce congestion there. Practicing ejaculatory retention too long without emitting sperm or having orgasm is not only useless, it will also harm both partners (sperm nourishes the woman; to withhold it from her is in a sense to deprive her of food).

A more interesting and useful way of approaching the sex act is to study the opposition of energies. For if one's goal is sexual intensity, seminal retention is not the way to achieve it. Ultimately it leads to greater fatigue, in spite of the fact that no sperm has been emitted. As already explained, releasing sperm or vaginal fluids is not the only ways of losing *jing*.

It should also be pointed out that unleashing one's fantasies is not the same thing as achieving true sexual vitality, as the great Taiwanese Taoist master Huai-Chin Nan has noted. "Sexual manifestations are good signs of vitality," he says, "as long as one's daily meditations are not connected with sexual fantasies."

Meditation is a good way to maintain physical vigor and freedom of mind. Detachment from worldly conditions is indispensable for natural sexuality. Wild desires and erotic passions are never the signs of a healthy sexuality but are the beginning of physical and mental decay. Taoists believe that the ardors of the heart must be tempered by clarity of mind. "The fire of the heart," they say, in their symbolic language, "must be calmed by the water of the kidneys."

Huai-Chin Nan has also stressed the risks associated with

obstructing ejaculation, especially through pressure on the *huiyin* point, at the perineum:

> Some people are teaching how to apply pressure on certain acupuncture points to stop the emission of sperm. Those who learn these methods often become impotent. . . . Those who contaminate their blood by blocking ejaculation lose weight and acquire a yellow complexion.

Ekiken, from Japan, citing ancient Chinese sources, warns against seminal retention as well, from the standpoint of longevity:

> If, after the appearance of sexual desire and the excitation of the kidneys, one prevents oneself from ejaculating and does not discharge the energy, this same energy will cause obstruction in the lower abdomen, producing boils or tumors. These problems can be avoided by taking a hot bath and massaging the abdomen.

These remarks should not obscure the fact that there does exist a genuine science in this domain, but it is not accessible to everyone and necessarily requires the help of a master. Moreover, for Taoists it is not the principal path.

SUN SI-MIAO'S ADVICE ON MAKING LOVE

Here are a few general indications from the treatises of Sun Si-miao concerning the correct way to carry out the sex act:

> Before going to sleep, the partners should indulge in erotic play designed to excite their desire, so that they end up tenderly intertwined; otherwise, they will not find joy and harmony.
>
> While you are having sex, massage yourself so that *qi* will circulate, pay attention to your breathing, swallow your saliva (liquid of jade), focus your mind on your *dantian*, and breathe deeply into the abdomen.
>
> When you ejaculate, close your mouth, hold your breath, clench your fists, breathe through your nose, and then let your teeth clatter. All of these gestures are intended to reconstitute the sperm, revivify vital essence *(jing)*, and nourish and rest the brain.

METHOD FOR PROLONGING SEXUAL INTERCOURSE

Ejaculation just after penetration or before the woman reaches orgasm is called premature ejaculation. Complex Taoist *qigong* exercises address this problem through visualization techniques. These techniques bring into play considerable energies, and anyone wishing to use them must already be well versed in the practice of meditation. There is nothing erotic about these visualizations; on the contrary, their goal is to cool the flames of desire by working on the body's most subtle energies. They are therefore not for everyone, and here again only a qualified master can lead someone safely down this path.

And so, for informational purposes only, here is a description of one of these methods for controlling ejaculation, to be practiced only under expert guidance:

> The man should imagine a luminous red drop in his *dantian*, just below the navel, golden within and red with white stripes on the outside. He should imagine this essence divided into two halves, a sun and a moon, which move apart from each other within this region and rise up to a point at the base of his brain where the two halves reunite.
>
> All the while, his penis should be at rest in the woman's body, as he drinks his saliva and absorbs his sexual secretions. The moment that he feels his sperm moving and he is ready to ejaculate, he must withdraw his penis. Only expert Taoists can accomplish this. The *dantian* is located just below the navel, and the center of the head is located at the back of the skull at the level of the eyes.
>
> He must imagine the shape of a sun (the *dantian*) and of a moon (the center of the head), about three thumb widths in diameter, joined together into a single shape. It is what is called the sun and the moon joined in a tight bond. Concentrating on this image during sex can be very beneficial.

THE NUMBER NINE

The ancient Taoist masters described a method that allows prolonged sexual intercourse without relying on ejaculatory obstruction. This technique, or "Great Yang" method, is based on energy laws and on the *I Ching*. These principles are the same ones that guide traditional acupuncturists, who tone *qi* by turning or moving the needle nine times. In the method described below, the principle is the same, but here the penis is the "needle."

The "Jade Wand" can be moved in nine different ways:

First, to the right and to the left, as a warrior uses a beam to break apart enemy forces;

then up and down, like a wild horse jumping across a mountain stream;

then like a flock of seagulls playing above the waves, darting in and out;

then with light pecks and deep thrusts in alternation, like a bird searching for grains of rice among grains of earth;

then with light thrusts interspersed with deep but slow penetrations, like stones thrown into the sea, sinking slowly;

then penetrating slowly, like a serpent slinking into his nest as winter approaches;

then penetrating quickly, quivering all the while, like a frightened rat scurrying into his burrow;

then penetrating gently, the way one might drag one's feet or as an eagle holds a rabbit in its talons;

and finally, lifting back your head and diving down, like the sail of a boat beneath the gale.

THE DRAGON POSITIONS

Apart from its erotic aspects, the art of Japanese and Chinese prints serves pedagogical purposes; its goal is not so much to arouse the imaginations of the sexual partners—which rarely require stimulation—as to provide the lovers with necessary technical details. In the past these drawings have formed an integral part of Taoist sexological treatises. There are many methods and systems of lovemaking positions, all of which have aspects that are at the same time hygienic, therapeutic, spiritual, and erotic.

The positions presented here derive from the treatise of the Woman of Purity. The positions correspond to the eight trigrams of the *I Ching*. Each of its four yang and four yin trigrams corresponds to a beneficial lovemaking position. Each of these therapeutic lovemaking positions corresponds to a different energy channel, reflecting the Taoists' observation that by stimulating these channels one can correct the imbalances—changes in the muscles, breathing, energy and blood circulation, glandular secretions—associated with them.

This art of lovemaking can also be regarded as a kind of sexual yoga. The Indian tantric tradition is a famous example. In these positions, the woman takes the role of natural and placid initiator; while the man concentrates on restraining his orgasm, she lets herself go, and as she gives her energies to him, she also receives the cosmic forces. The strength that one derives from these therapeutic positions is proportional to the degree of the man's concentration and the free circulation of the woman's curative energies.

Taoist texts and treatises mention many sexual positions: one of these ancient treatises contains more than 120. It is not the sheer number of these positions or even their acrobatism that makes them interesting; nor is it their aesthetic or sensual aims. The important thing about these exercises is their profound effect on the *qi* of their practitioners.

These positions act on certain zones of the penis and the vagina, which can be described as energy zones. These reflexology zones, which few people know about, are indicated in the figures below. Just as with the ear or the hand, in the sexual organs every part is linked to one of the body's major internal organs.

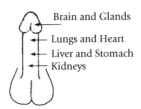

Brain and Glands
Lungs and Heart
Liver and Stomach
Kidneys

Energy zones of the penis.

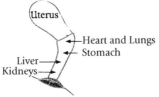

Uterus
Heart and Lungs
Stomach
Liver
Kidneys

Energy zones of the vagina.

These positions are not for everyone. People's sexual organs fit together in different ways, and this, combined with a lack of flexibility in the partners' bodies, can make certain movements impossible.

We will now explain in detail the major positions; some are useful in improving the energies of men, while others are tonics for women. It cannot be overemphasized that these positions are an integral part of the sexual Tao and are not to be practiced for the sake of mere sensual diversion.

Position 1

Lying on her side, the woman spreads her thighs as wide as she can. While she is in this position, the man practices the nine methods (see above) for ten to fifteen minutes.

This position is particularly effective for toning sexual energy and remedying certain sexual deficiencies, such as partial impotence in the man or inhibited orgasm in the woman.

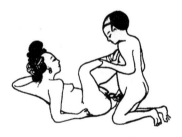

The Dragon turns over.

Position 2

This is a simple position. The woman lies across a large pillow so that her lower back is curved and her sexual organ is tilted slightly upward. The man practices the nine methods over a period of fifteen days.

This position is a complete *qi* energy tonic for both partners. It is also considered a stimulant for the five *zang* organs, or viscera—the liver, heart, spleen, lungs, and kidneys—particularly for the woman.

Position 3

This position is very well known. The woman is in a kneeling position and remains nearly still. The man has the active role, as he moves his pelvis up and down. As with the previous position, this position should be practiced over the course of a fifteen-day period to really activate the energy process.

This exercise is beneficial in cases of deficiency of blood, anemia, poor blood circulation, and low blood pressure. Chinese medicine would say that this position eliminates the blood stases that are at the source of many health problems.

Position 4

This position is particularly good for women. The woman lies down and wraps her legs around the man. Note that her legs encircle his thighs, not his waist. The man should not penetrate deeply in this position; he should not create intense pressure.

This position stimulates primarily the woman's digestive organs—the liver, gall bladder, and spleen. It also improves the distribution of energy in the joints and relieves aches and pains.

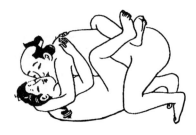

ONE DEEP AND NINE LIGHT

Some aspects of this Taoist technique are already known in the West. This method uses the penis as an acupuncture needle, that is, to tone *qi*.

It consists of a sort of rhythmic massage that is done during sex. In one of the positions listed below, the man begins with nine light, superficial penetrations followed by one deeper penetration. Then he makes eight light penetrations followed by two deep penetrations, and so on, according to the following sequence:

ORDER	SHALLOW YANG THRUSTS	DEEP YIN THRUSTS
1	9	1
2	8	2
3	7	3
4	6	4
5	5	5
6	4	6
7	3	7
8	2	8
9	1	9

Once the man has completed this cycle without ejaculating, he can begin it again.

This method improves control of ejaculation and makes for perfect stimulation. It also permits complete stimulation of a number of the zones of the penis and the vagina that correspond to the most important internal organs. This method, used in combination with the preceding ones, will enhance their effectiveness.

SEX AND SPIRITUAL REALIZATION

THE FUSION OF YIN AND YANG

Attaining higher levels of consciousness through natural means has always been the goal or aspiration of Taoists. There are many natural ways to facilitate spiritual expansion and the attainment of harmony: breathing, meditation, contemplation of nature (without obsessional reveries, of course), art (nonerotic painting, music, dance), the healing arts (Tai Chi Chuan, *qigong, daoyin*), the martial arts and warrior ecstasies such as kung fu and strategy (with all due reservations regarding these latter "arts," geared as they are to the taking of human life—Taoists have tended to be crafty diplomats, not fanatic samurais), and, of course, the practice of sex, which, as a method of spiritual attainment, was often criticized by the moralistic Confucianists and their modern descendants.

Sex, like art, joy, birth, illness, and death, is one of life's supreme—and supremely powerful—experiences; that is why complete awareness during the sex act can bring about contact with the primordial world, the energy- and consciousness-filled precognitive universe that is the Tao (which some call the "divine"). What is sex, after all, if not the spontaneous manifestation of *qi*? *Qi* is universal energy, both subtle and marvelous. It fills the universe and accomplishes various functions, some of them subtle, others not. In sum, every force, every energy, is a manifestation of *qi*: the circulation of blood, the forces of gravity, attraction, and repulsion.

Though invisible, *qi* governs the physiological functions and participates in many aspects of the sex act, coordinating the different organs and functions—the sexual organs, blood circulation, the secretion of natural fluids, sensory stimulation, the emission of sperm, sensations—in a variety of ways. All these functions depend on the proper circulation of *qi* through the network of channels, in the blood, and throughout the nervous system. The quality of *qi* is thus extremely important for consciousness.

Sex can be different things: It can be a purely mechanical performance or the spontaneous accomplishment of a natural act. When a person is aroused by a film or a fantasy, the desire engendered in him is a pseudodesire. If he acts on this desire, the result is nothing more than a mechanical performance, dictated by a desire that, whether consciously or not, is a purely mental construct. On the other hand, when your sex organ awakens naturally in the middle of the night and you fulfill your natural sexual inclination, you are accomplishing a natural act and replenishing yourself with *qi*.

This way of looking at things may seem paradoxical to a Westerner, given that many contemporary schools of psy-

chotherapy encourage fantasy through their "talking cures."
Let there be no mistake, however: Taoism is not the way
of fantasy and dreams but the path of objective truth and
enlightened consciousness.

Taoists are of the firm conviction that natural spontaneity is not a commonly encountered human behavioral
trait. From this perspective, regaining spontaneity means
searching for a state of consciousness in which there are no
preconceived ideas, a natural state unencumbered by life-
negating thoughts. So often we revel, simply by force of
habit, in our melancholy and even morbidity. Sometimes
we adopt narrow-minded attitudes and postures of sadness
and defend these states vehemently, insisting that we have
a right to be sad or feel angry.

Spontaneity of that sort is limited indeed and affects
more than our behavior. We must therefore go beyond
these appearances and look for the origin of our behavior
to see if we can't find a less conditioned source.

That source is the spontaneity of our deep inner nature.
Here, too, the practice of meditation turns out to be necessary. As Lao-tzu said, "Original nature can produce all
experiences. Original nature is the essence of spontaneous
goodness. To be natural in one's actions is to always be
pure and calm."

One might thus conclude that to act spontaneously is to
behave in a manner appropriate to the present situation
with complete sincerity and without malice. This spontaneity seems nearly identical to what we call deep intuition.
Without this quality and without nonaction, it is hard to
open the energy channels. As the proverb says, "One can't
make grass grow by pulling on it!"

As for our daily lives, we often wonder why our minds are so weak, so inconsistent. The Taoists have an answer: when we indiscriminately follow the path of attachment to objects of desire, we weaken *shen*. The philosophy of non-action is thus far from representing an anything-goes lifestyle.

A treatise by Huai Nanzi sums it up this way: "When one uses one's consciousness day after day, it moves farther and farther away. It attaches itself to the object of desire and is incapable of returning to man's center." It also seems that on this level the energy of consciousness is attuned to the body's other energies. As the *Taiping Jingchao* notes,

The energies of the body circulate around it, above it, and below it. The essence of consciousness uses these energies to enter the body and to leave it. When these energies are depleted, the spirit disperses and withdraws, like the fish that dies when the water has dried up.

SEXUALITY AND HUMAN EMOTIONS

The romantic feelings, the artificial desires, and the unquenchable thirst for experience that present-day society engenders in us are a source more of internal conflict than of freedom in the area of sexuality. The earliest Taoist texts stress the destructive effects of uncontrolled emotions. The old sage Lao-tzu, with his distrust of the five tastes, the five sounds, and the five colors, always kept his distance from sensorial perceptions and the attachments they create. The lines of

Lu Dong Bing are as invaluable as ever in helping us understand the phenomenon of conflictual emotions:

> Because man has six organs, he develops six consciousnesses and thus six emotions. People do not realize that their emotions keep essential reality hidden from them. And it is when one loses sight of essential reality that the emotions run wild. The root cause of the negative emotions is envy, however. Thus, if you are not dominated by your desires, you will not be irresistibly attracted by things, and if you are not attracted, you will not be disgusted by other things and anger will not be born. And without anger there is neither fear nor sadness.

Other Taoists speak of these emotions as poisons that not only cause conflicts with others but also obstruct the flow of vital energy in very specific ways, resulting in loss of energy, constriction, and stress. It's commonly recognized that anger can raise blood pressure to dangerous levels and that hysterical joy can provoke a heart attack. If these are simply the most glaring manifestations, how many less visible obstructions must there be that little by little imprison the ego in a web of illusion?

It is also common knowledge that many chronic illnesses can be aggravated or even caused in the first place by these emotional obstructions. The way to recovery thus involves a second stage, that of freeing the emotional energies and redirecting them into the functional circuit of *qi*. It is not really spiritual work but rather a foundation for spiritual work. Many methods in this book work directly or indirectly on the alchemy of the emotions. The path to ridding oneself of these conflicts is simple: one has merely to see that there is no self, at least no real self. How does one become aware of this? By practicing contemplation and meditation. Lu Dong Bing compares the self to a shadow floating in space like the morning mist. How can illness take root in such a shadow? The basic advice on how to manage one's emotions is as follows: "Sit calmly *(Tso wang)* and observe the emotions rise just as you might watch the morning mist dissipate into the blue sky."

The conflictual emotions create numerous obstacles in us, as much on the physical, organic level as on the social level. The Taoists associated the principal emotions with the cycle of the five phases and the five viscera. This inspired notion allowed them to understand the phenomenon of psychosomatic illnesses long before the term had been invented. They did this by examining the seven emotions *(qi qing)* and considering their relation to the functioning of *qi*:

- Anger provokes a contraction of *qi* that affects the sinews (causing stress) and the liver.
- Sadness and remorse provoke loss of *qi* and chronic fatigue. Lung function is also affected.
- Anxiety and fear provoke a collapse of *qi* that damages the kidneys.
- Melancholy brings stagnation of *qi*, which obstructs the free functioning of the spleen and stomach.
- Envy provokes constriction that is akin to anger.
- Resentment blocks the expression of energy in the region of the heart.
- Impulsive joy and hysteria excite the heart and can weaken it to the point of fragility.

This brief description shows that for Taoists the body, energy, and consciousness are intimately linked and that people can become the slaves of their emotions and fall ill as a result. Their freedom thus becomes an illusion. How, then, can one say that emotional self-indulgence is freedom?

People are emotional beings; they are deeply sensitive to what happens around them and are always involving themselves, sometimes unwittingly, in complicated relationships. They want to be happy, but their happiness rests on a sweet illusion. They welcome life's good sides and stubbornly refuse to face up to its difficult moments. If the extreme emotions can so easily cause us to lose our balance, then how can we look on our emotions as clouds moving across the sky? The Taoists' response to this question is that we must make the attempt and practice as often as we can. In the beginning, this process seems intellectual, but visualization *(tzi)* and the cultivation of quietude give this method a natural force.

In China today, certain *qigong* methods are practiced with the aim of producing emotional release or violent upheaval. Many of these practices have no basis in traditional Taoist methodology. What's more, some of these schools have fallen under the sway of Western psychotherapy. Dr. Pang Heming, director of the Zhi Neng Qigong Hospital, objects to these practices in the strongest possible terms: "In China, many people practice *qigong* and experience episodes of uncontrollable screaming, crying, shaking, and many other so-called paranormal phenomena. This merely proves their total lack of a solid foundation. These illusory events are taken as signs of real progress."

The term "quietude" ought not be understood as a negative state excluding all sensorial or emotional stimuli.
On the contrary, quietude means a calm acceptance, free
from all conflictual emotion. As the Chinese proverb says,
"From an ounce of confusion comes a ton of chaos."
Solutions come more easily when the spirit is calm and
clear than when it is under the influence of impulsive,
violent emotions. That is the meaning of Taoist wis-
dom.

You cannot approach the Tao if your spirit lacks clarity
or if you are enslaved by your emotions. The teachings of
Lao-tzu express the touchstone role of the conflictual emotions. These teachings are one of the major themes of the
interior practice of Taoist transformation. Energy wasted on
worldly emotions is not at all useful in the great Taoist
purification process.

To put this advice in a modern framework, we might say
that stress binds up our vital energy in superfluous tensions, and violent emotions cloud our awareness, shroud-
ing it in extenuating circumstances that divert it from what
is essential. Envy, at the heart of our emotions, is for Taoists the source of all attachments; this thirst to possess, to
see, and to feel is, they believe, yin in nature, and thus
passive. It is a golden prison in which we believe we act
freely. In the *Tao-te Ching*, Lao-tzu expresses this idea for
us in a dazzling way: "In absolute quietude, how can desire
be born? When avidity remains unborn, that is the state of
absolute quietude."

This quietude is in fact a source of inexhaustible energy.
That is why the ancient sages would withdraw to the mountains, not to savor the simple joys of country life but to

partake in the beatifying calm of their own spirit washed clean of all vulgar attachments.

The same is true for your body and its sexual essence. Every morning, sexual essence grows within your body, and if you use it at the right moment, you will not harm yourself at all; the next time you use it, it will be even stronger: "Man misuses the sex act, sometimes even forcing himself when nature does not necessarily demand it."

SEX, PURITY, AND FREEDOM

Purity, in the Taoist sense of the term, is a state of freedom from all illusions, a state beyond the self, beyond heaven, and beyond earth. Impurity is the worldly way, the way of illusory attachments to endless desires. As the "immortal golden treatise" says, "The energy that begins to move when one attains quietude is ancestral energy *(yuanqi).* When *yuanqi* moves, *jing* increases. At this moment one can observe its proper nature. Even while remaining calm, one can guide *jing* to the *dantian* and create the alchemical pearl *(dan)."*

To be alive is necessarily to be in contact with the world, and thus involved in a never-ending production of thoughts and feelings. For the Taoists, worldly thoughts give rise to impure consciousness, to the loss of the original state. This original state is not at all one of hedonistic idleness or beatific torpor, because non-forgetfulness is there to awaken us at every step on the path that is the Tao.

To practice quietude is to return to the source of consciousness through meditation: when the eyes, the ears, and the five senses are no longer in contact with the world, they cease to trigger memories in the conscious heart (*xin*). As Confucius (K'ung Ch'iu) himself said, "When the desires diminish, the way to heaven is open."

Within the human body there exist many involuntary movements: the heart is a prime example. Action, for its part, conforms to the objective world conditioned by our thought. Nonaction is unconditioned. To free ourselves from the negative imprinting we bear in our bodies and our thoughts, Taoists offer the practice of meditation and contemplation. Every time we decide to act, we are conditioned by the weight of our memories and desires, even though it seems to us that we are acting of our own free will. For example, if we decide to take a vacation in a warm, sunny place, we believe that in making that choice we are acting in complete freedom. In fact, if we examine our motivations, we perceive that our action is conditioned by different subjective points of view: our stress and fatigue, our desire to get to know one more country, a thirst for human encounters to relieve our loneliness, the current fashions that make this destination obligatory, and so on. Our act, far from being free, is in fact preconditioned. What we call freedom of action is often more like a golden prison. The practice of nonaction thus consists of finding our way back to the state that lies at the very heart of our physical and mental being.

He Xiugu, "the little long-stemmed lotus flower," was the only woman among the eight immortals of the Taoist pantheon. As a child, she had already attained immortality and awakening, and she thereupon took vows of chastity. When her stepmother wanted to force her to marry, she fled to the celestial regions, "leaving her shoes behind her." Once there, she was asked whether she didn't miss the world of men and women, of lovers and their mistresses. This is how she answered: "My friends, the immortals, possess the qualities of both sexes."